I Awake to Another Day...

Finding the Light with Multiple Sclerosis

By

Frederick L. Keller

Table of Contents

Introduction:

This book is a first-hand account of my journey with Multiple Sclerosis (MS). As I went through the stages of diagnosis to disease management, it became apparent that while there were numerous books written on the subject of MS, most focused on the medical or clinical aspects of the disease. While these sources were certainly empirically informative, they were coldly lacking in the emotional preparation and guidance that I needed. There is a profoundly personal side to any life-changing diagnosis, and this is where the true struggle resided for me. I couldn't turn to anything of a nonclinical substance that would help guide me through the emotional and mental turmoil I was experiencing. There was so much I wanted to know not only from my doctors, but also from other people with MS. As I started navigating my way through things in a bit of a clumsy fashion, I was inspired to write down my thoughts and insight as that new person with MS and what they would likely want to know not only about the disease but also about themselves. This book covers the time I reflected over the year leading up to my diagnosis and the first year after receiving my diagnosis with MS.

The book is divided into three distinct parts. Part One looks at a wide variety of personal topics and experiences and the impact Multiple Sclerosis has played on each. There are times of frustration, denial and sorrow. There are topics of extreme support and heroes that have stepped up in my journey. There are character traits that can be of benefit and others that can be detrimental. The intent has been to capture these aspects, feelings and thought-provoking situations and how MS has touched it all. In a way, this section is a reflection of my own personal struggle through the initial blow of learning about my MS and coming to accept it as a part of who I now am.

Part Two focuses on moving from a position of understanding to truly accepting what MS means in my life. Acceptance doesn't just mean sitting still, but gaining a clear mind on how you are going to choose to live with MS. Acceptance is not just formed from the perspective of being that someone with MS, but it is formed by the people around me as well. Friends, coworkers, and family all will be affected by this disease in some way, and it is vitally important that we prepare to help everyone touched by MS come to a pure sense of acceptance.

Part Three is all about capitalizing on the sense of acceptance and beginning to focus on those specific efforts and the needed energy to beat it. Knowing there is no cure today does not mean that I just give up. There are so many things that can be done to maintain a "normal" life, but it takes work and a proactive frame of mind. Like many struggles we can all face in our lives, MS is really no different. There is almost always a way to make a situation like this better, but it does take time, effort, and determination.

From a personal perspective, this book intends to do two things…to help others better understand the everyday experiences of a person with MS, to know what the disease takes away, and also what the disease gives. The second, to help me as a person with MS move beyond merely accepting this disease and knowing that regardless of what limitations I may end up with, that I can contribute to a better result, a brighter future for someone, be a better father and husband to my family, and look back and feel good about my life…every minute of it. Life can be so much more if I can find the way to live with MS in my life rather than find a way to fit my life into MS. My wish to the second point is that it will do the same for you.

Part One: Discovery, Denial and Understanding

Chapter 1: What Exactly is MS?

I do not prescribe to be a doctor so my attempt is only to pass along the facts that I have been communicated not only by the doctors I have spoken with but the vast array of published and documented clinical evidence and information that is available to anyone on the subject. Multiple Sclerosis (MS) is thought to be an auto immune disease. Quite simply, it is thought to be a disease where the body attacks the central nervous system. This attack ultimately causes sclerosis or scarring that resides in and on the nervous system. As a result and over time, the body ultimately succumbs to this scarring whereby damage can be permanent leaving behind reduced function of the body's ability to transmit signals down the nerve pathways. The damage can vary depending on the severity of the sclerosis.

MS is a progressive disease. While there are four known types of MS, they all seem to have a similar and fundamental purpose to attack the nervous system. Where they basically differ is in their speed, frequency and state of damage over time. There are an estimated two million people in the world that have been diagnosed with MS and roughly 400,000 in the U.S. Each week over 200 people are diagnosed in the U.S. with the disease. This equates to roughly one person every hour of every day that is diagnosed with Multiple Sclerosis.

There is no definitive test that a doctor can give you to determine if you have MS. It is generally a hard disease to diagnose because of this fact. In most cases, there are a series of tests that are initially performed to baseline if someone may have MS. These include MRI scans and studies of the brain and spinal column to look for sclerotic activity generally referred to as lesions. There are neurological tests such as an evoked response test to look at nerve conductivity, signal speed and interruptions in nerve transmission.

And finally there is a lumbar puncture where a small amount of spinal fluid is drawn and evaluated for oligoclonal bands or an increase in certain antibodies that is an indication of increased immune activity in the spinal fluid.

In conjunction with these tests there are currently two basic criteria followed for diagnosing MS. The first is the person must have had at least two relapses or episodes where symptoms are present which must be at least a month apart. The second is there must be more than one lesion on the brain or spinal cord. As you can see from just this limited information, the diagnosis can be complex and time consuming.

As differing as things can be in the diagnosis process for so many, so too are the symptoms that MS patients experience. The simple fact with MS is that because the damage can manifest itself differently in various parts of the nervous system across different patients, it will almost undoubtedly yield different symptoms. For one patient it may mean problems walking. For another patient it may mean difficulty swallowing or seeing. I'm not certain if the statistic is a clinical opinion or fact, but I have been told by several doctors that there are over fifty "typical" symptoms related to MS.

For most people, learning they have MS is in many ways a relief. I know it was for me. There was not so much a sense of joy in learning I had it, but knowing that I had MS allowed me to stop wondering what was wrong and move on to dealing with it. The road that an MS patient will travel is long. It is bumpy and treacherous at times…but it can be traveled.

Chapter 2: Reflecting on My Diagnosis

I remember waking up as a seven or eight year old the day after Christmas having that feeling of excitement realizing I had a new toy; a remote controlled car. Just thinking about all the fun I was going to have and how excited I was seemed incredible; it was my whole world. Even when I wasn't playing with it, I was thinking about playing with it. I then recall being a little older and the excitement of waking up in the morning for my baseball game. My Little League team was the Braves. I planned what I was going to do; how I was going to bat and how good I was going to play. I thought about the win and what it would feel like. The thought consumed me just as the remote controlled car did.

When I got even a little older…during my teenage years…it was all about driving. Just wondering what it was going to be like was almost unbearable. The morning came and I woke up ready to take my driver's test knowing that freedom was just within reach…assuming I passed.

I wish so many times I could have mornings like that again. I love my life…don't get me wrong. I love my family and all they give me. There is tremendous excitement and joy that I get from having great kids and a super wife. But there was something very different about the way I use to experience things for myself that is very different now. There are things that consume me now and it's not just things related to growing up and getting older or becoming more responsible. There are things in my life now that I have absolutely no control over. Things I would have never thought about waking up to on any morning.

A morning for me now generally consists of waking up and lying there for a minute trying not to move too much and focusing on feeling normal. It almost takes me to a point where I wonder maybe it's gone away, but then I have to move. I am reminded rather quickly that no…in fact it is still here with me. So…I get on out of bed and start the day…without that long remembered "start". It's a very different day. No more remote control car. No more wins on the baseball field except maybe for that first minute just lying there. Just wishing and wanting something different.

Looking back now over the years, I remember several symptoms that come to mind...several events and situations where I didn't feel right. Not too long after we bought our motor home, I remember taking our family on a trip to a state park. The trip wasn't anything too intense just a weekend getaway. We had gone on a short walk near a small river that ran through the park and after getting back to the motor home, I remember sitting there at the table realizing that my back was numb up and down my spine. Of course I didn't really think too much of it. In fact, someone like me simply dismisses it. It must be stress or maybe the way I walked on the hike...something. And then there were other things that started to happen as I reflect back on them now. My balance was starting to falter. Fingers and toes began going numb. If I closed my eyes for a few seconds, I literally could not account for where my feet were. Small tremors started happening. All of these things I again chalked up to stress or nerves…maybe too much going on at work. Whatever the case may be, I'm the kind of person that finds it pretty easy to come up with some other reason, other than a medical reason, to explain why something must be happening to me. And so this is how the disease really started for me…founded in denial. Maybe denial isn't the right word because to deny something means you have to admit it exists. I certainly wasn't going to do that. And it is only now that I can look back and realize how much I overlooked.

By the spring of 2009, I knew things weren't right. The numbness I had experienced in my back was now rather pronounced. Other symptoms came with it now…pins and needles…other sharp or piercing pains, numbness in other parts of my arms and extremities. I was having difficulty feeling sensations such as hot or cold. Tremors and muscle spasms became a daily event. Many of them became debilitating and would stop me in my tracks regardless of what I was doing. The fact that I was experiencing these things and couldn't figure out why was constantly on my mind. I couldn't move through this mentally much less physically. I had never experienced anything quite like this in my entire life. And to make such a statement is rather profound given my experiences. I was a daring individual most of my life. I have broken many bones over the years doing "crazy" things as my parents would say. Snowboarding glaciers, cliff jumping, racing bikes, sky diving, you name it; I did it. I was also involved in a rather serious car accident during my high school years…no, I wasn't driving like most would expect the teenager to be at fault…but rather was a passenger as my mom drove me to school one day on an icy winter morning. The soft top Jeep we were in hit a patch of ice, she lost control, and we were flipped into a telephone pole. We both suffered serious injuries including punctured lungs, bruised kidneys, broken ribs, arms and fingers. Point being I am no stranger to my body breaking and the aches and pains of life. But one thing I can say about all these other events that set this event apart…I healed from everything before…but I couldn't find the same this time.

This disease is very different; it's silent and unknown. It makes me think about it harder. It stays on my mind…fresh and up front in a much more intense way over any other thought I have experienced. I'm an individual that will search for a reason as to why. I have always asked the right questions in my mind, but I couldn't come up with an answer. Maybe there wasn't a why; it just exists.

It really didn't start to sink in that I had Multiple Sclerosis until August 2009. I had gone through all the testing and had all sorts of neurological issues. I guess it wasn't until I started to literally see it in print, maybe from a doctor's note or from an MRI reading, that I began to realize what this really meant. I was just starting to travel a new road. It was a road where there wasn't an easy answer. No way was this happening to me.

I am coming up close to my anniversary date of officially being diagnosed. I've learned quite a bit about this disease over the past year. There are so many questions to ask and answer. How does this disease work? What does it do to people? Who has it? Is it a progressive disease or will I wake up in another month and be confined to a wheelchair? Who can I talk to? How do I deal with all this? What about the other aspects of the disease that I can't read about. Why does MS affect people differently? I sit in the doctor's office and see the full spectrum of folks from those that look "normal" to those that are confined to wheelchairs and need help to do just about everything. All of these people share the same thing…we all have MS.

Chapter 3: Playing Catch

I look at pictures of a time when I was maybe five or six. I had a makeshift uniform on a t-ball team with the iron-on letters that spelled "Stingrays". There is a picture of a small, skinny boy with a floppy red helmet on (likely several sizes too big) swinging a bat at a ball on a tee. Next picture is rounding first…then second…then third…and finally in to home. I can honestly say I don't remember that specific event, but I do remember the time and other memories from my t-ball experience. I remember how proud I was to almost effortlessly catch the ball. It's a big deal for a little boy to learn how to catch. We almost all have the innate ability to throw things, but to catch something takes an entirely different set of skills. I recall the only real meaningful "miss" I ever experienced while playing catch which occurred a couple of years later. I wasn't paying attention during warm ups, and the ball hit me square in the mouth splitting my lower lip wide open. It ended up not being a terrible split, but I could still stick my tongue in the gash and push both pieces apart.

Now when I am asked to play catch, it is generally with one of my kids. They have it down, and I still feel like the youngster of five or six learning all over again. I can't even play anymore without thinking I'm going to get another split lip and not because I am not paying attention, but because I literally can't get my glove in the right place to catch the ball. Multiple Sclerosis has severely impaired my hand eye coordination. I do not have a genuine sense of where my hand actually is to start with and then to have my brain tell my hand where it should be seems to cause all sorts of issues. The end result...I look like I never learned to catch a baseball in the first place. My reaction to move to the ball...to get the glove positioned...to watch the ball into my glove and to close down on the catch is choppy and delayed causing almost a spastic type of reaction with my catching arm and hand. If I catch the ball, it is more often by luck. I'm fortunate my kids are still pretty young and cannot throw that hard with twins that are eleven and a seven year old, so if I do get hit in the lip again, it shouldn't split it too badly.

To take such a simple and almost effortless activity that I struggle to perform and put it in the context of other more complex activities that I would expect myself to do as an adult scares me to even try and imagine. I don't know if it is over thinking or what…but my mind goes absolutely in a million directions with no resolve. This one…simple…childish accomplishment…is the epitome of what I now nearly 35 years later strive to reach.

Chapter 4: Woodworking

This is my hobby gone wild! I have been engulfed in woodworking for many years, and I have the equipment and tools to prove it. I have a father that is and always has been extremely inclined to dabble in this particular area and coupled with his mechanical and engineering approach he taught me quite a bit when I was younger. His father was a master craftsman in a time when woodworking was truly a work of art. Hand tools ruled his day and powered tools were in their infancy. I remember helping out on many different projects my dad undertook and having a distinct interest in how things came together…how he approached a particular challenge and "engineered" a solution. I even today have the very furniture my grandfather made for my dad when he was a boy. It was passed down to me, and I have passed it on to my two boys.

The intensity for woodworking really came to me after I married in my late twenties. Not sure exactly why…but when it took, there was no turning back. I was infatuated with building anything and everything. Woodworking is a very personal hobby because so much of it is done in your head before you ever touch the wood. It is just as an artist approaches their masterpiece. Form takes shape from an inner vision, and all of it has to come together through a very deliberate manipulation. Joinery, reading the grain and patterning pieces so they match or compliment each other, fitting with precise exactness and having the patience to bring it all to an inspiring conclusion are all a part of the woodworking process. It can be exhausting…consuming…perfectly satisfying. And the woodworker has to be up to the task. Projects involving large pieces such as furniture or artful pieces can take weeks or months from start to finish. There have been times I was so engulfed in a project that I found myself turning on saws and other power tools well past 2:00am! Even when I did come to bed, I would lay there for hours thinking about the next cut I needed to make and how I was going to approach it to make sure it was perfect.

All of this can take a toll on anyone. One may think that a hobby such as woodworking can't be all that physical; I assure you it absolutely is. The skills and muscles you call upon to do the plethora of tasks involved in any project are immense. And in all this excitement and anxiousness to create, I noticed an ever so slight shake in my right hand. Particularly the harder I tried to steady my hand the more difficult it became and the intensity of the shaking increased. If I stopped trying…the shaking would stop. It was so weird and not in a million years would I have imagined at that point what was in store for me in my nearest future.

One of the most important mental capacities you have to possess to be a successful and accomplished woodworker is confidence. You must be confident in your skills…not arrogant…but to have the ability to know that you can call upon your physical skills to accomplish what you have envisioned in your mind. It is imperative to take your woodworking to new levels. At some point soon after MS took a foothold in my life, I lost a great deal of my confidence. It has impacted me in ways I pray I will be able to overcome even if I am never able to physically get past this disease. I want more than anything to get it back. Over the past year, I haven't done much woodworking at all...mainly because I can't get past the mental handicap I now possess in losing my confidence. I can absolutely understand now how people who lose something or someone so close to them come to the crossroads of simply giving up.

Chapter 5: The Handicap Placard

I'll bet most people have either joked about it themselves or heard someone else joking about it...the frustration of having to pass up that "oh so precious" parking spot up front. You almost "wish" for a second you had some ailment that qualified you to park there. What a perk that would be; to realize no matter what establishment you pull up to and because of this great country we live in, you could have the right to park in your own spot! Think of the time you could save. Think of the damage you would avoid to your vehicle. What an absolute convenience if I only had that placard.

I joke about it, but I will admit that I have most certainly thought about this as a desired luxury more than once in my life...almost coveting those that are part of this elite group. Not that I want any of the baggage that goes along with getting the privileged parking place, but it would be awesome to get the perks.

I didn't think about that parking spot too much after I started having my own issues. I guess I was preoccupied with the unselfish reality of having a genuine health problem. How could I have been so thoughtless and dismissive? Disabled people have earned the right to get that spot and how dare I envy and joke about their benefit as though it was something they won, and I didn't. I'm ashamed for that.

It wasn't until about six months after being diagnosed that I started to question my own ability to function to my own set of "normal" standards. That included all the mobility and recreation that falls within these standards. One of my more difficult situations to address is all the misfires that seem to occur when I have to walk for any period of time. It seems to start with my balance. Because my balance is off, I am very unsure of my footing most times. In addition, I also have numbness and muscle spasms/contractions in my feet and legs. My foot could be numb almost entirely and with the balance issues, I have the ingredients for a good fall if I'm not careful. Tack on to that a hot day or a long distance to walk and fatigue sets in extremely fast. I don't mean just feeling tired. I mean feeling so physically spent that you literally expect your body to collapse.

Fatigue that requires you to stop everything you are doing then and there and rest. It sometimes takes hours or days to recover.

Take this situation and a simple task like going to the grocery store on a busy day and you could be parking quite a ways from the store. I have experienced the hardship of literally not being able to walk due to my MS, and it leaves quite an impression on your mind. It runs through my head as I have to start off across the asphalt. I walk past that vacant handicap spot now and the reality of my situation hits me right between the eyes. I'm wishing and praying that the day never comes that I have to park there.

In May of 2010 after taking my family to a local rodeo, I almost didn't make it into the arena. Later that month I succumbed to the reality of my disability and had my wife take care of getting me a permanent handicap placard; I wasn't even able to do it myself. It wasn't the MS that kept me from going in to the DMV on my own; it was my pride. I'm still apprehensive to use the placard. They say part of the acceptance process is denial. All I know is I would trade just about anything to be assigned the farthest parking spot in any lot every day for what it took to get the parking privilege of that handicap placard.

Chapter 6: Eating

This is one of those past times that after the age of two or three you think you pretty much have it down. You may not have the "manners" that your parents feel you should possess, but the fact that you can use a fork and spoon (given most parents probably aren't going to let a two or three year old have a knife) is a huge milestone. The act of eating has never really been seen as an art in my family although it has definitely been a passion. It is such a natural part of my life just like breathing or sleeping. It's another one of those things I have always taken for granted.

When I started to notice my tremor, I not only noticed it when I was trying to do intricate tasks with woodworking, but I also blaringly noticed it when I would attempt to eat. Just the slightest tremor with a fork full of peas and you are likely not going to get any of them to your mouth. It sounds a little funny, but after a while it can turn furthest from. Because my hands not only tremor but at times feel numb, I lose the touch to even pick up the simplest of foods with a utensil. I would tirelessly try and just get more and more frustrated. I would get downright mad with myself. There is no other way to describe it.

Eating would turn to such frustration that I would even snap at my family when they were simply trying to talk to me at mealtime. The difficulty in performing the simple function of feeding myself would quickly turn to a self conscious event. It felt like everyone was looking at me.   And why wouldn't they as it looked like I have some problem. I know if it were me looking at the same situation I would think the person was on drugs or something. Take this situation to the professional level and now I am seated at a business dinner. Now it becomes more than just personal. I have to be on; I can't have something like this happen now. How will this affect what people think? How will this affect my career?

I would have never imagined such a ridiculous situation would cause me to question how this disability could affect my future work opportunities, but it did and does. Do I just break down and tell everyone what is going on when it happens? I have done a pretty good job hiding my MS for quite some time but as the physical effects of MS have started to settle in and take hold of my physical capabilities, I have to find a way to let people know. I feel I owe it to them and owe it to myself. But that is easier said than done.

What falls off my fork or the fact that I cannot hold a utensil properly because I can't feel my fingers has brought me to a point where I don't know how to get past it. There are so many frustrating inconveniences with MS. There are things that create personal situations that I have no idea how to handle or deal with. Never in a million years would I have thought I would be contemplating how to explain to my family, friends or coworkers why I sometimes eat like a two year old. Why I have to bring my head down to my fork or spoon in fear of dropping everything. Why I end up scooping food into my mouth.

My pride makes it near impossible to find the best way to have that conversation. I realize I need to spend more time thinking about how to deliver the message and be prepared with the conversation that will likely transpire thereafter. Not only for others, but so I can get past it myself.

Chapter 7: Working

If you think how hard it could be for someone to hide things from their families or friends then how much harder...or easier...would it be to hide something from coworkers? I say hide because it seemed like such a natural reaction to hide my MS at work. I not only wanted to hide from my job, but also from my dignity, self worth and of course the disease. Maybe then it wouldn't find me.

I guess I became most self conscious about MS at work. It bothered me and still does what people think about me. It is a very self-preserving sentiment I know, but I am being honest. What would coworkers think if they saw me stumble or lose my balance? What would they say about me if they saw a bad day when I was riddled with continual tremors? What would I do if a muscle cramp or contraction came on me while I was in an important meeting or better yet when I was in front of a hundred people giving a presentation?

At first, symptoms were somewhat easy to hide. Because MS is a progressive disease, symptoms start off rather subtle. The first symptom I remember hiding was my tremor. I historically have eaten lunch with my teammates. I am in charge of several teams of people and I have coached to them and believed myself for years that an open and exchange rich environment fosters collaboration and success. Just trying to get a bottle of water to my mouth without shaking was a feat. In fact, it became impossible. As days and months went on, my tremor became worse and more pronounced. Even though the medications I was taking to reduce my tremor would help, the disease always seemed to stay one step ahead.

It finally got to a point where I labored to find the best way to break the news to my team. I talked about it over several conversations with my wife and continued to avoid the topic for many days…maybe even weeks. But I had to do it. That was one of the toughest moments so far with MS. These were people who depended on me for their livelihood. I know my family depended on me and I on them, but this was different. This was about their ability to count on me as a leader, and I felt that by sharing my MS with them that I was somehow letting them down; I somehow felt less of a leader.

I remember sitting down in one of our conference rooms surrounded by all the teams I lead after calling an impromptu meeting. They were a bit on edge as impromptu meetings aren't terribly popular at my work. I started off by telling them about some of my past medical issues and trying to explain what they may have seen. In the end, I told them that I had been diagnosed with MS. It was really the first time I had heard myself say it publicly. It was very awkward and unnatural, but it was a start to what I knew I would be dealing with for the rest of my life or until a cure is found.

One thing is for certain; true character is rarely called to the charge in times of static calmness, but is most evident in times of dynamic turmoil. I can't say it any more succinctly than my team rallied around me. They encouraged me and comforted me. They prayed for me and believed in me. They reinforced their sentiment that despite what I had told them, they still trusted me to lead.

My symptoms have progressed even further since I delivered the news, and my coworkers and teammates have a better understanding of what MS brings to the office. While I honestly still hold some desire to hide at times, I know that I work with a great group of people who stand by and with me. While there is no way I can or even want to wear the "sandwich board" of MS to everyone I meet at work, there is comfort in the place I have reached at this point with my MS at work.

Chapter 8: Losing Senses

To go along with my visible symptoms to date which primarily center on balance and coordination issues, tremors, muscle contractions and spasms, I also experience on a periodic basis strange hot or cold sensations in different parts of my body. These generally seem to happen in my upper back near my neck and my arms down into my wrists. It's hard to explain as it doesn't feel like something hot or something cold is touching you from the outside, rather it feels like something from the inside. I noticed it at first wearing a watch with a metal band.

I continually was looking down at my wrist at work. It felt as though something hot was coming out of my arm from under my watch. I couldn't tell if it was my watch, so I took it off and had someone else feel it to see…maybe it was heating up or something was wrong with it. Not at all…it was me. For some reason it was as if my body was sensing the metal band all wrong and telling my brain that it was something hot. It ended up distracting me so much that I had to stop wearing the watch and switched to one with a leather band.

It happens more frequently in warmer weather for me, and it can be an extreme sense of cold or hot. It's a little scary as I don't know how intense it will get, and I have no way of stopping it. Since there isn't really anything external that is producing the hot or cold feeling, it can make for an awkward situation with the folks around me.

The other sense depravity that I experience is numbness. It generally gets worse during a relapse or after exerting myself or when I get tired, but there is a perpetual numbness to a large extent that I have in parts of my hands and feet, which is scary. Not so much that I can go numb because I think most people have experienced short term numbness from something they did. Maybe they slept on their arm funny or stayed in a particular position too long. The scary part of the numbness for me resides in the fact that it can be dangerous. I have burned myself and even cut myself, and I didn't even know it. I recall one time recently I was doing some electrical work on an outlet and had a utility knife in my hand to strip some wire. Apparently I didn't realize that as the knife slipped off the wire sheathing I had pulled it across two fingers. I didn't even realize it until I saw blood on the wall and the outlet box and looked down to discover what I had done.

I have also burned myself and not felt a thing. It could be that I touched something like a grill that I thought would have been cooled off only to realize that the gas was still on and because I wasn't looking directly at it with my eyes at the time and was moving too quickly, I ended up touching the grate and walked away with second degree burns. My wife constantly has to remind me to be careful around the kitchen whether it's a warning from touching something hot or worrying about me cutting myself with a knife. I guess it's a bigger deal to my family than I realize. For me, the bigger deal is knowing I may not ever have the senses I did before MS. What will I do if more of my sense of feeling goes away? How hard will it be to completely lose my sense of feeling or touch and still function? This is one of those "I don't want to think about it" MS problems that rank

right up there with not being able to walk.

Chapter 9: Impact on My Kids

I have fraternal twins (boy and girl) that turn twelve this November, as well as a seven year old boy. Like any other proud parent I have no hesitation to say they are the best kids a father could have. They certainly have their moments like any other parent would likely say, but I love them with all I've got and take nothing for granted about the impression I as their dad leave behind. For good or for bad every day is a lesson taught whether I like it or not. I don't mean to leave my wife out of this train of thought, but I want to focus on my kids first as the discovery process is quite different for kids. I will leave my wife for a separate reflection.

I remember my wife and I talking about what it would be like to have kids. In our discussions they were always about "the good times" that we would have. We never reflected on someone getting sick or hurt. It wasn't out of ignorance or naivety that we avoided the thought, it was simply our inner desire to focus on what could be and all the good that could come with it.

When I started having issues, I kept it from my kids almost as well as I kept it from people at work. My exhaustion was most evident at times, but they really didn't think too much of it...or so I thought. They would ask me to do things with them and sometimes I could while other times I couldn't. I guess it was easier for them since they had siblings to turn to if dad couldn't step up to the task. Other symptoms were more difficult to hide, but I just passed it off as being tired.

After a while though, it was clear they knew something wasn't right. The biggest problem didn't seem to be that particular point but the fact that I hadn't told them the truth. I remember my wife and I finally sitting down with them and explaining to them what was wrong with me. We timed telling them after we had informed the grandparents for fear they may say something prematurely in an awkward moment. I don't even know if we used the words Multiple Sclerosis in that initial conversation. We explained that I had a problem with my muscles and nerves. That my nerves weren't working the way they were supposed to, and they weren't telling my body what to do. We talked about some of the things they may have seen such as the tremors or me cringing when a muscle contraction was at its worst.

It looked like while they understood what we were telling them, they had other questions they just weren't asking. I guess something like this can't be talked about all in one sitting. And so we have had a few other discussions when the moment arose, sometimes with all three of them together…sometimes individually. They know more about MS now although it is all age-appropriate knowledge. There is so much more I feel I owe them though. In time I will need to find how best to share the entirety of how MS is a part of my life. In reflecting back to those days of my wife and I "dreaming" about what it would be like with kids, we now have to weave into our family thread a disease that has struck the heart of our home. I hope they will understand and someday know that despite what MS has taken away from me and the opportunities it has robbed from us as a family to do certain things together, that I would have done things differently if I were able.

Chapter 10: My First Relapse

I had heard of the progressive and remittent characteristics of MS but had never really experienced them for myself with any definitive delineation until October 2009. I certainly had symptoms and sometimes they were more intense than others but for the most part things were manageable. The word relapse had been mentioned but only in passing conversations with my neurologist. It was never used in context to anything directly related to my MS.

I know enough to tell you that all MS patients experience things differently. Not all neurological damage is done in the same manner and to the same degree, so our experiences with symptoms and debilitations can widely vary. It is also not to say that every MS patient experiences things completely different. I know a number of MS patients that have numbness and muscle spasms in various parts of their body.

The rush of pain and muscle cramps was overwhelming. As I mentioned earlier, I am no stranger to physical pain in my life. I have had three shoulder surgeries, survived a major car accident as a teenager and have broken many bones over the years. This was completely different. It was as though MS was lurking in the shadows waiting for me to be distracted before it would hit me hard. My joints hurt as if they had been beaten. I could hardly walk. My ankles, knees, hips, wrists, elbows were all affected. I was fatigued beyond clear thought. I was as close to bedridden as I had ever been for several weeks. I had help from my neurologist, but there was no miracle pill or drug to take to make this go away. I could get some alleviation for a short period of time, but the MS had to play out its hand.

I can't tell you how furious I became at my MS. I had thought I was fighting a pretty good fight up until then. Maybe I was even a bit arrogant towards my MS. Maybe it took advantage of my guard being down and my taking it for granted. At any rate, in the aftermath of my first relapse, I ironically felt closer to my MS.

I still have issues today as a result of my first relapse. My knees and hips are less flexible. They don't "respond" as well as they had in the past. I have a great deal of joint popping and swelling at times. My tremors and muscle contractions can be much more pronounced particularly when I grow tired or fatigued. I keep looking for the day I will wake up and declare that I have fully recovered from that first relapse; it hasn't come yet.

I have a great deal of respect for veteran MS patients. Many of them have gone through a multitude of relapses and still hold their hopes and spirits high. While I find my own way through the light and shadows knowing that there are other relapses waiting for me in time, I look to my first experience to help me through the next.

Chapter 11: The Doctor that Helps is the Doctor that Listens

Having worked in the healthcare field for nearly twenty years now, it is amazing how different managing our healthcare is today than when I was a child. I remember going to the doctor to get shots and when I was sick, but never do I recall my parents questioning the doctor. If the doctor said I had something or we needed to do this or do that…we did it with no question or concern. There was an assumed trust and expectation that your doctor always had the answer. And not that he or she had just an answer, but they possessed the right answer.

I certainly do not want to imply that doctors today are less capable than they were years ago, but our involvement in our own personal healthcare has immensely changed. I know for myself I have certainly been more involved in my healthcare decisions with my doctor but never as much as when I was diagnosed with MS. My first experience with a neurologist wasn't actually all that great. I had gone at the suggestion of my family doctor whom I trust and have known for over ten years now. After all the testing and follow up, he actually said he didn't know what was wrong. I couldn't believe it! If it had been like when I was a child, I would have simply walked out of that office and assumed that it must all be in my head.

But I knew better. MS is not an easy diagnosis. There isn't a one-test-fits-all to find out. In fact, it seems that many MS patients go through a great deal of stress and medical tribulation before they find out what is really going on. This is why some who have MS don't get accurately diagnosed for quite some time. Not all neurologists are trained to identify much less work with MS patients. So I kept looking for an answer. I remember a comment in passing that a doctor friend once told me that means more to me today than ever, "If you are going to a doctor that is trying but can't find a way to help you, then it's time to find a new doctor."

Knowing what I know now about Multiple Sclerosis, to catch this disease in its early stages is absolutely critical. More damage can be done in the first two to three years of the disease than in the next ten. I see older patients in the doctor's office that have had MS for twenty or thirty years and didn't have any real treatment options when they were originally diagnosed. The fact that they missed the early window of treatment certainly had an impact on the progression of the disease and sitting there watching them struggle to walk, or move, or see is enough to convince me all over again that taking control of your medical fate and getting involved in the medical avenues you will need to travel is imperative. In fact, I know that it has given me back some quality time.

My own personal tenacity is only a testimony to the fact that when you do find a great and understanding neurologist, I suggest you stick with them. MS is a two-fold disease. There is the actual neurological damage that is present and then there are all the symptoms caused by the damage. My doctor is exceptional not only because of his medical skill set, but because he listens to what I tell him. He listens to what my symptoms tell him. He is open and expects me to be involved in my care. He also knows that listening helps me to better manage this disease. The fact that I stayed strong in my search for an answer is a testament to the new age we all as patients need to play in our medical futures.

Chapter 12: Remember?

I know the saying that as you get older your memory goes…though I have always hoped that if this were the case for me that it would happen when I was very old and people would expect it of me. Maybe I would even have my kids or grandkids around me to help me out, and it wouldn't be such a big deal. I know that I struggle with watching my parents or my wife's parents "forget" things, but it seems rather harmless. It isn't like they are forgetting to take their medicine or forgetting how to get home from the grocery store. It is generally characterized with forgetfulness to recollect…likely a memory or not finishing a sentence because they are thinking of too many things at that time.

Memory loss for me is one of those MS symptoms that seem much scarier to contemplate experiencing. To not be able to accomplish something physically is one thing because more often than not there are other ways to skin the cat. With your memory though there is no substitute. There is nothing to take its place.

I haven't said much to my family, but I have started to experience problems with my memory. It has been harmless to this point, but it is such a helpless feeling when it happens. Most of my experiences have been when I am very tired, but I seem to forget short term events that may have just happened in the past day or so. Maybe it was something I did or something I talked to someone about. Alcohol can make it worse. In fact, I don't even drink anymore except at home under supervision…not that I do it regularly at all.

I have been experiencing memory issues at work and at home. I can be walking down a hallway at work and after a few steps I literally have forgotten what I was going to do. I stand there for a moment and then go back to my office. For the life of me I cannot remember what I was walking down that hall to do. It has happened more and more in the recent months. I can be in a meeting and talking about a particular subject and just forget mid sentence what I was saying. This wasn't supposed to happen until I was eighty…

If physical limitations add to a self conscious complex and to lack of confidence then adding memory loss on top of it seems darn near impossible to overcome. What else can this disease dole out? I worry that this type of limitation could be devastating to my family in terms of compromising my job, leaving my kids with someone less than a dad, or becoming an untenable burden on my wife. I try every day to make sure MS doesn't take the focus of my existence away, but it is hard. What will make this effort even worse is not being able to remember whether I won or lost.

Chapter 13: Steroids

This is an MS patient's nirvana. I relate the immediate benefits of steroids to that of an anesthesiologist when you are having surgery. They take away the pain and leave you in a different place where you can escape the symptoms of this disease. It is generally short lived, but steroids for me can get me back in front of my MS…ahead of the game so to speak.

I remember taking my first round of steroids actually a few months before I was diagnosed. I had been experiencing several symptoms and some were increasing in severity. Steroids are almost euphoric. The dose that you receive over a two-to-three-day regimen is extremely high…not like a steroid pack you may get when you have a sinus infection. These doses are much, much higher. They are delivered intravenously, and all I can say is they make me feel like I was twenty again. There is no better way to describe it. Within hours and sometimes even minutes after completing an infusion, symptoms that could have been bothering me for days or weeks are reduced to near nothing. I have not had great luck in getting steroid infusions to eliminate my tremors, but they definitely help with my walking, my joints and balance issues, my agility and stamina and my overall sense of being more than I was before the infusion. They mentally make me feel much more alert and energized maybe even to the point of fooling my brain into thinking I could do just about anything.

I can see why these things are protected as a controlled substance. I can also see how athletes can become addicted to such an enhancing substance. I remember the staff warning me that many people who get steroid infusions have a dominant and immediate side effect of tasting metal in their mouth. They offered me gum and candy, but I thought I would give it a try without anything. In fact, I was a bit intrigued by the idea of tasting metal in my mouth. I thought it would be a little neat to at least experience it.

I never had the metal taste, but I had no problem eating the candy and treats they provided. The steroid rounds brought me a sense of hope. While there isn't a cure, there is an escape and at times when you are suffering from debilitating and painful symptoms that escape is a godsend. It's enough.

I have had two other steroid infusions over the past year and a half, and each time they have been very helpful. The long term impact though is enough that you cannot count on them on a regular basis. Bone density issues and other osteoporotic problems along with heart conditions can become prevalent from overuse of steroids. You hear the stories of people who abuse steroids in a recreational fashion and the issues they have…well, many of them are indeed true and even in a controlled and legally administered fashion, they have their drawbacks.

But they are a valuable weapon in the arsenal to fight this disease. I will admit some days I wish I could go in and get another infusion just like I was deciding to stop and get fast food. Maybe it would help with a bad day or get me back on track from some rough and persistent symptoms. Yet I have come to realize that the steroids are my crutch for now that I can lean on from time to time. They will certainly help to prop me up, however; they are not a solution by themselves that will get me to where I need to go.

Chapter 14: The Farm House

Nearly two years ago my wife and I decided to dive head first into a dream we have had for over a decade. We had purchased an historical home some time back before we had kids and renovated a good portion of it over a three year period up until the time we had our twins. Now remodeling is not woodworking, so while I was doing constructive types of things there is a whole new world involved in remodeling. I certainly enjoyed the experience, and we knew my knowledge of woodworking would come in handy some day in the future; this was our chance.

My wife has always been great at searching out real estate. If you give her some specs to go from, she will certainly find you what you were looking for. And so she did. With nearly eight acres and a small farmhouse in a rural part of Williamson County, Tennessee, it was a sight for sore eyes. It wasn't that old, but the home needed a ton of TLC. We both had a vision and saw through all of the muck and outdated fixtures. The immediate yard around the house probably had five years worth of trash around it. There was a mountain of work to be done.

When you have ambition, your health and dedication, you can make great strides on fulfilling a small dream like remodeling an entire farm house. I don't mean putting in a few new lights and painting; I'm talking about ripping out the entire home down to the studs, moving walls, creating new space, reworking plumbing and all the electrical and then moving on to all the finish work , cabinetry, flooring, everything.

We had made great strides. We worked tirelessly and even got our kids into the groove with helping out. We cleaned up the entire outside of the property. There were acres of debris, trash and dilapidated outbuildings. We had ripped out all the old inside the house and reworked all the new walls and rooms, electrical and plumbing. We installed all the drywall. We were on our way to looking like a successful DIY series.

When I started having my issues with MS, the first thing I remember working on our farm house was the fatigue that set in. I lost so much of my drive and energy to keep pace. I remember trying to lay tile in a newly installed shower one day, and I completed about three rows of tile work; I was absolutely exhausted. I had to stop. I literally could not do anymore. I was so disappointed with myself. I was ashamed and viewed my efforts as simply pathetic.

That was over a year ago, and we are still working on the house today. We are nearing completion of the interior, but there is still a great deal of work to be done. The project has almost become a physical rendition of my inner struggle. It is huge and formidable. I have to work on it in stages and take it a piece at a time. I have good days and I have bad days. But the remodel is actually helping me to cope with this disease. We look to the end of the project, and my wife and I wonder what it will be like. We see the newness of everything and how wonderful it will be.

But it is hard…harder than I ever would have imagined. Not the work itself, but the "mentalness" of it all. The fact that I continue to put myself in a situation to test my own limitations which I know to be shorter than they were before MS and all the while realizing that I will somehow have to find a way to ultimately get this project completed. There is no quitting. There is no failing. There is only a driven individual and family…a shared dream…and the feeling of what it will be like when everything is finished…new…and fixed. The farm house truly does remind me of my struggle and echoes my battle with MS.

Chapter 15: Adrenaline

What a natural drug…and it is absolutely great. It ranks right up there with steroids but in a more "personalized" way. I have always had fun optimizing my own production of this stuff. I don't know if there is a limit to the amount of adrenaline you can experience, but I am fairly certain I have reached my personal potential over the years. I have done quite a bit in my life to get the "a" factory in full production. I started snowboarding when I was in high school. This was back in the 80's when snowboarding wasn't even known. I remember finally getting access to a local mountain in western Massachusetts with a buddy of mine, and we had to show them that snowboarding was, at a minimum, safe and nonintrusive to other skiers. I remember how it made me feel and the rush…the pure rush…I got from doing it. There was nothing else like it.

It was one of the freest feelings I had ever had. It opened my visual horizon of what I was able to do. Up until then I had stuck to traditional sports such as baseball or soccer, and I was pretty good at getting the knack. But now I was in what felt like my natural element. This sport consumed me. I spent a great deal of my time around snowboarding. I even started a company, incorporated and all, at age 18. A buddy and I ultimately turned it into a lesson-based program that we had at two local ski resorts. It worked out great.

You can't buy that kind of feeling though...the rush...feeling invincible. It only comes with certain circumstances or events in life. I have snowboarded the best places across this nation from Colorado to New Mexico to Wyoming to Salt Lake City to Banff. I have been on trails and out of bounds. I have been on extreme cliffs and dropped over thirty feet in freefall on a sixty-degree slope. I have been launched inverted on a nine-foot-high natural snow drift on Peak 7 at Breckenridge with a professional photographer...and have the pics to prove it. I attended the University of Colorado at Boulder as a full-time student for three days a week and was a full-time snowboarder for four days a week. And I did this every week and every year of college.

When you experience such a feeling…such a rush of life…you never are far from wanting it again. It doesn't matter how old you are or how far you are from where you experienced it. You will want that feeling again. I believe if I could get it back I could conquer anything… including this inconvenience called MS. When I could summon my adrenaline potential at will and harness its capability, I was invincible. I broke bones and laughed it off.

So how do I get from where I am now to that same feeling? It's kind of like finding the missing pieces of a puzzle I guess. I would recognize them if I saw them…know their shape and intended fit…but I have to know where to look and recognize what I am looking at. MS affords you no insight. It seeks out adrenaline just as I have over the years. It is as though I am competing with it for what my body can produce. It has robbed me of my potential and will certainly try and steal from me again. I have to find out how to beat it at its own game…and win.

Chapter 16: My Wife

I reflected earlier on the impact to my kids and felt I owed an entirely separate reflection for my wife. Not because the impact of MS is any less for her than it is for my kids but rather she deserves way more than I can give her without this disease much less with it. We have been married for fourteen years, she is my best friend. I count on her and she counts on me.

Like so many husbands, I am a fix-it man. If my wife comes to me with a problem, I naturally try to fix it. Most of the time though she just wants me to listen and not do anything. Even after so many years, I still don't have this down. It just doesn't feel natural to me to not try. It makes me feel so much more of a man to know I can help to fix something when it is broken.

I sense one of the most troublesome fears for my wife is losing me. I don't say this because I think too much of myself, but I see the way she looks on the outside and imagine how she feels on the inside when the subject has been discussed. Truth is I'm just as scared when

I think about losing her even though I know I don't show it the same way she does.

She has always been so strong through this entire ordeal. From the very beginning when I started having symptoms and issues through the diagnosis and even today, she has always been the positive anchor for both of us. So many times I have been frustrated or angry at my MS, but she always helps to pull me back to a brighter center.

I don't know what it would be like if I had to go through this alone. I can't even imagine it quite honestly. And with this very statement is an irony of my situation. If I were going through this alone, then I wouldn't have to deal with the thought of letting someone down because of my MS. In my mind of being there to "fix it", I am literally plagued with a debilitation that one day will likely not allow me to fix it. My personal worth to my family is partly rooted in my capabilities…at least in my mind. If my capabilities are diminished, how much more then is my personal worth diminished as well. I know it sounds crazy, but I am bothered by this fact more than I am bothered by what MS could potentially do to me. I simply cannot let my family down.

And this is where my wife steps in and changes the tempo. She lifts me up with her encouragement and her own sheer determination to never give up on me. She is that coach every kid should have that tells you "You can!" We have been through a lot together. From delivering nearly thirteen pounds of babies at one time to suffering a pulmonary embolism and nearly losing her, she and I were meant to be. If doing this all over with her meant knowing I would get MS all over again, I would not hesitate to take that dive.

In the end, maybe it won't be so bad if I can't be the fix-it man I once was. My wife is more than capable of being the fix-it woman.

Chapter 17: How to Fight

I've wondered many times how best do I go about dealing with all this? Do I look to a better diet? Is there a specific exercise routine I should do? Maybe I should move to a different climate? What books do I read first? It is exhausting and overwhelming to know where to begin, much less figuring out how this is all going to work...if it will even work. And by work I simply mean help.

I will start by saying I learned a great deal from the National MS Society. Even before I was diagnosed, my doctor told me to learn what I could about some of the more common neurological disorders that plague so many. This certainly included MS. The information the National MS Society provides takes you from ground zero telling you about the symptoms and the various treatment options to the current research that is being done. It points you in the right direction for certain.

Fact is because this is a progressive disease, there are possibly years ahead of dealing with different symptoms or certainly different degrees of the same symptoms. When you throw this fact into the mix, it can make managing MS much more difficult. What you do today to deal with a particular symptom or issue may not be the same way to deal with it in five years. This fact is the same for other physical issues as well, such as high blood pressure or diabetes.

Since being diagnosed and even more recently since my first relapse, I have started listening to my body much more. I know there is a point of no return where stress, physical exertion, heat or lack of sleep can take me to the edge. This edge that I am referring to isn't just an edge of exhaustion. It is a point at which there is an exponential degradation of my symptoms. Once this occurs, it can start a chain reaction that inside of a few hours or days could throw me into another relapse. In many ways, symptoms can lie almost dormant until all the right ingredients are there to make them explode. You have to learn what ingredients are specific to your point of no return.

I have tried exercising, but this is a slippery slope for me. Not everyone has this issue, but I naturally can work up a sweat with little effort. My body heat can rise relatively fast and this is not good for my MS. In addition, I tend to work out in a more than moderate approach and this ends up tasking my muscles beyond what they can take. After a few times of exercising, I end up behind the curve of recovering where waiting until I actually feel better doesn't do my workout schedule any good, so I end up pushing myself to the point of no return. My next alternative will be to give swimming a try. At least here I should be able to keep my body temperature in check and still get a good physical and cardiovascular workout.

The other extreme: not exercising is just as bad. When you sit around and do nothing, you build up atrophic muscles. I can become very stiff and sometimes even have my joints swell because they are getting no use. It's funny how the ingredients in my point of no return can be at opposite ends of the spectrum, but they can. And I consider myself somewhat lucky as I don't have other health issues of any significance that I have to deal with. For some, MS is but one of their limitations.

I have to admit that even today I haven't figured it all out. As I said before I have good days, and I have bad days. My doctor once said the first goal to realize is to simply be able to reflect and know that you have had more good days than bad days. I guess this is where I am at in my fight. One thing is for certain; the fight means nothing without being prepared and however long that takes, I will take it. I want to know that when my time comes and I have to fight this disease with all I have that I am at least able to say that I did everything I could to win.

Chapter 18: Taking Shots

I know I don't have it nearly as bad as say someone with diabetes, but then again my situation isn't too far from. When I started evaluating the different MS treatment options...and there are several...it came down to accepting the fact that regardless of which option I was going to choose, it was going to involve giving myself a shot if not every day then at least every other day. While there are other treatment options that involve monthly or yearly infusions, these were not the best options for me. I'm not going to say that one MS treatment is better than another. There are many MS patients that I have spoken to that over time have even had to change treatment medications. One treatment may no longer provide the benefits needed while there is another therapy that maybe in the beginning didn't do them any good now benefits them greatly.

I am on my first injection therapy and have been for nearly a year now. The inconvenience of giving myself a shot isn't all that bad. I'm not a terribly "fatty" person so finding adequate places to give myself an injection is a bit challenging. Most of the time I end up giving myself shots in my stomach area. It's hard to believe that I may have to do this the rest of my life. If I do the simple math and just assume I live another forty years, then I will have given myself more than 7,250 shots. Each shot costs about $125 so over the next forty years, I will have tallied up over $900,000 in just shots! Not that I have to pay for them in their entirety, but still.

It shouldn't be a financial question for me, but because I have been in healthcare for nearly twenty years now and most of my career has been focusing on the cost components of healthcare, I cannot help but to think every time I mix up my injection and get ready for my shot how much money I feel I am potentially wasting to the healthcare system of this country. And then I start to get mad at the entire situation all over again. Maybe it is a good reminder that I have to take a shot every other day, so that I can get re-grounded in what all this means.

My advice to anyone who has recently been diagnosed with MS or to someone who has a friend or family member who has recently been diagnosed with MS...don't wait one day to start your treatment! The damage MS does during the first two years is the greatest and the detriment that waiting to start any therapy can have to a newly diagnosed patient is not something you will want to think back on in five or ten years and wish you could do over. After my nine-month follow up and seeing my MRI scans, I am convinced that the therapies offered can absolutely help. Even if they buy me three or five quality years, it will be worth it. To think back to my financial scenario, even if the cost for those three or five years was the entire $900,000, and I had to pay for all of it myself, I would try and find a way. It's easy for anyone to say there is no way three or even five years would be worth that...but anyone who answers that question in that way doesn't have to live with MS.

Chapter 19: Dancing

This is a subject that is bound to get me into trouble with my wife. For starters, I literally don't believe I can remember one time when I have actually danced with my wife. Unbelievable I know, but true nonetheless. To explain how I ended up in this situation and then the added luck of my outlook starts back when I was very young.

I remember growing up with parents who enjoyed life. Both of my parents worked which wasn't terribly common back in the 1970's. I started coming home from school on my own to an empty house in the third grade and would go grab our hidden key in the back yard. Letting myself in, I would stay around the house until my parents came home from work. Today this would likely get them turned in to the authorities by a nosey neighbor, but then it was a great freedom and responsibility I took seriously and enjoyed. I don't see any issues with it and wish I had the guts to do the same with my kids today.

At any rate, when the weekends came, my parents loved to go out and have a good time. Many of those times they would go out dancing with friends. They would get me and eventually me and my sister a baby sitter and we all would have our own little "night out" so to speak. Special events would come up, and we all would be out...many times dancing. I guess I never really saw the fun in it for myself because I was a kid and always wanted to be doing something else. I would sometimes get dragged out to dance with someone and never really liked it all that much.

Maybe it carried over into adulthood or maybe I just considered myself a bad dancer. Whatever the case, I never really had the desire to nor did I consider it at all cool to go dancing. When I met my wife, we didn't date for terribly long before we were engaged and ultimately married. At our wedding, we had a simple ceremony and a quick reception after...no dancing. Even at our rehearsal dinner the evening before...no dancing. We talked about it at times after we were married, and I know my wife looked forward to it. She even would subtly ask me at times over the years if I was interested in taking a class. Of course I would remember what it was like for me as a child and would quickly give my "we'll see" answer.

With some of my MS-related issues today, I literally don't know if I could even do it now. With my balance being terrible and poor hand-eye coordination, I guess I'm afraid I won't be any good. I would hate to ruin it for her after she has looked forward to it for over fourteen years now. I sure do wish I could take back at least one of those "we'll see" answers. So many simple yet reflectively satisfying items on the list of life remain for us to do together like dancing. It's funny the little things that you think about when you fear that you won't ever be able to experience them again. Half of the people who are diagnosed with MS within fifteen years can no longer walk. That is enough motivation to get out there and dance.

Chapter 20: Heating Up

While most of my MS symptoms are generated from the disease itself, there is one external factor that seems to have a dramatic effect on all of my symptoms. For many MS patients this same exacerbating reality exists. When core temperature starts to rise above normal, it produces an amplified effect on many MS-related symptoms. While many times my core temperature can rise due to physical exertion such as working out even in a temperature-controlled environment, it can also rise with simple everyday tasks when the outside temperature and/or humidity are high.

For my own experience, both heat and humidity independent of each other and certainly together have a dramatic impact on my symptoms. For one, my energy level is significantly reduced on hot or humid days. It is almost as if you stuck a hole in the bottom of a barrel and the water drained out. That is how quickly my energy can escape me. Behind the energy drain is usually increasing muscle cramps not only in frequency but also in severity. Some cramps are incapacitating.

Weird sensations of pins and needles, cold and hot, the feeling of something touching me, dagger-like sensations, even numbness are amplified the higher my core body temperature increases. If it gets too high, then it could tip me over the edge and either renders me impaired for days or weeks with certain symptoms becoming exponentially worsened, or for some people, it can throw them into relapse. I have not experienced the latter myself, but now that I have this disease, I can certainly see this happening if I am not careful.

In middle Tennessee the summers can be not only hot but also humid. Come the middle of July, temperatures can easily reach into the mid 90's and with the humidity it can produce relative temperatures well above 110. Doing something as simple as trying to mow a small yard can be a serious hazard. I remember one day this past summer trying to help my wife mow the yard at a farm we own out in the country. I could barely make a lap…maybe two…before I had to literally go inside and get in not only the air conditioning but also sit in front of a floor fan for quite some time just to cool down.

I can feel myself slipping into the hands of my disease when I get overheated. I have started to become much more aware of how MS works specifically on my body and when it is time to change my direction or effort to avoid spiraling downward. It is a very delicate balance in the summertime between the things I want or need to do and how I allocate and break up the time needed to perform each one. And how I would go about doing a similar task in the winter time when I don't have the external factors at least to worry about is very different.

It is a bit ironic that the sensation of heat cannot be felt by my finer sense of touch say in my hand or certain fingers, meaning I cannot necessarily tell that I am getting burned, but the same "sense" when represented differently...say in the weather...can have a profound impact on my entire physical disposition.

Chapter 21: My Sister

We try and stay in touch, but I don't do everything I need to in keeping up my relationship with my sister. She lives over seven hours away, so visits are few and far between. We both have the hectic lives of parents and working way too much. But I have no excuse. We are nearly six years apart in age and like any brother and sister we grew up having our glimpses of getting along and not getting along. I certainly wish now I had been a better brother.

With our age difference, we never had friends that we shared and never shared any space in school together. By the time I was in high school she was still in elementary or middle school and by the time I graduated she was still a year from starting high school. I have always loved my sister, but I know that I didn't show her much respect when we were younger.

That is certainly different now. She earned a scholarship for college. She has done well with her career. She is the mother of great children and made me an uncle two times over. She has accomplished a great deal in her life and has a wonderful family she is very proud of. I am so very proud of all she has become.

While our time spent together is not near what I want it to be, we talk frequently and try to get our families together at least a few times a year. This past summer during our normal get-together on the Fourth of July, my sister gave me a gift…one that I will never forget. She gave me a DVD that had on it a short presentation of her, a friend and her youngest son participating in an MS walk. They had participated in it earlier that year and sported homemade t-shirts that proclaimed "Beat MS". There were so many people there, and I know it wasn't easy to show up on a cold morning with a four year old and commit to walk. Her friend…best friend from my knowing…also walked.

As I watched the video she made for me, I was overwhelmed with a strong sense of pride. She had done this for me and took a stand to fight what was plaguing me. While I am still trying to find out how all this fits in my life and what to make of it, she has stepped into the middle of it all and rolled up her sleeves. She has helped to inspire me to do more for myself, my family and for my MS.

I hope she knows how much I love and respect her. I also know I owe her so much…not for the things she has given me over the past but what she has given me for the future. She has given me a sense of hope and vigor. I am not only compelled but driven to fight harder. If she can show up as she did on a cold winter morning to walk for me, then I should in the very least fight knowing I have family behind me that loves and cares for me. When all is said and done, that is one of the richest feelings I will have.

Chapter 22: Faith

If you ask most people what faith means to them they more than likely will tell you what they believe. I would say that for most of my life I would have answered the same. My intentions here are not to persuade you to believe what I believe in terms of a religious or spiritual position. That quite honestly is between you and God. I would rather use the term faith to look inward and ask you to test it for yourself. With MS, you will almost certainly come to face this at some point along the journey.

I once heard a great pastor at our church speak on faith, and I think it applies not only to our spiritual lives but also our physical lives. He said that faith is a combination of three things: Belief, Trust and Action. You see belief alone doesn't really describe your level of faith…not entirely. I can believe what someone is telling me based on the facts they are stating, but that doesn't mean that I trust them or that I will act on their words. And through faith we weed through not only what we believe, but then what we choose to trust in and ultimately act on. All of these together indicate our level of faith. When you act on something daily, trust and believe in it daily, then it clearly means more to you than any one of these three things on their own.

Now, I probably have you wondering what all this has to do with MS? Am I saying that a person should have faith in MS as a disease? It is certainly real, so I believe it is there. It is trustworthy in the sense that I know it will be there tomorrow and trust it to do what I know it can do and it forces me to act each and every day. I must have "faith" in MS…right? I guess if the epicenter of my relationship with this disease was the MS itself, then it would seem that my faith would logically be placed here.

But turning this on edge a bit and keeping myself at the epicenter of my relationship with this disease paints an entirely different picture of what I have faith in. Remember, faith is a result of what I believe, trust and will act on. You could say that MS is yet another thing that has entered my life that I have to deal with as it has for thousands of others. How I embrace it and relate to it is ultimately up to me...no one else.

What I learn about MS for me personally has shaped what I believe I can do in the face of MS. Learning to trust myself in the face of MS is taking time. Trust in my body and in my mind to be there physically when I need it is a hard hurdle to clear knowing this disease can rob me of my own inner trust and cause me to doubt what is possible. But these two pieces of the faith puzzle, belief and trust, move me to act. To act not only for my own selfish interest, but for my wife, kids, father, mother and all those that have this disease that maybe didn't get an opportunity to act; this is part of my charge. I don't know why I have MS or how I got it, but that is not the faith question to ask.

The faith question starts and stops with knowing that I now have it and what impact it will have on my life. How will MS help to shape what I have faith in? How can I be a better person through this experience? While I personally would prescribe that the only way to have physical success in the fight against MS is to start with a solid spiritual faith foundation to build from, I expect to look back on this entire MS experience someday regardless of what it does to me physically and answer the question if asked "Do you have faith they will find a cure?" I will say without hesitation "Yes". As long as there are people who continue to believe in the effort, trust in their abilities, and act on what we know, then faith will most definitely lead us to the cure.

Chapter 23: Confidence

I touched on this in an earlier section on woodworking but wanted to spend more time on the subject as there is so much more to the dynamics at play regarding my confidence in my physical and mental capabilities. Confidence is such a precious trait to possess, but it has often been misinterpreted by so many including myself and has often been taken for granted.

My wife and I have always been conscientious about fostering a profound sense of self-confidence in our kids. There is such a delicate balance to it all. First, you can't act on things too early say with a toddler because they likely will not understand what it means. Wait too long and you miss the window to build on early events that start a youngster on a "winning" track to confidence through successful results. In many ways, it will be in a big part the way we measure our success as parents...by seeing how confident our kids are in themselves and the decisions they make in life.

As fragile as it is to nurture and grow, I never would have dreamt in a million years that after all the work that goes into fostering a strong sense of confidence and watching it blossom and mature, that someday it could be in jeopardy from something as silly as a limp or a twitch. But it can...and sadly for me it has been. I don't make this statement to get a sympathetic ear from my family or friends or coworkers. I say it because I know that admitting it is hopefully the start to getting it back. It is also amazing to me how quickly it can start to disappear. I first noticed it with my woodworking, but now it permeates through so many things for me.

Whether it is a work-related event or being around my in-laws or parents or my kids Boy Scout troop...anything where I can be seen for less than I know I used to be makes me feel vulnerable to losing more of my confidence. And for much of it, I feel like what it maybe took ten years to gain in confidence, say through promotions at work and increased responsibility and reliance from coworkers, can be literally gone after a couple of awkward moments.

This is one of the biggest problems I feel I face with MS. Not having the confidence I have experienced for most of my life means to me that I am a different person. I am somehow less of a person. It also means I am not the person I know I can be. This disease is constantly trying to rob me of my own identity, and if I'm not careful, it will selfishly take it all without looking back. Part of my reason for writing this book is to not lose sight of what is important in this battle. I have to constantly be willing to remind myself of this fact. I have to realize that just as I try to carefully manage the lessons of confidence for my kids, that the same applies to me and maybe even more so in the face of adversity.

Chapter 24: Prepping the RV

We are getting ready to go on a weekend reunion with my wife's side of the family and we have gone to get our motor home out of storage. We have had such great times with our RV. My wife and I talk about the days to come when we can travel on our own and go wherever we want to go. There is so much of this country that she longs to see, and I think it would be great for us to experience it together.

Yet getting the RV out of storage is also a sobering reminder of thoughts from over a year ago…in fact in a few months it will be coming up on two years…that I recall experiencing that initial numbing feeling in my back. I distinctly remember it as I sat at the table in the "kitchen-living-dining" room. It has become a permanent memory and is reinforced every time I step into that motor home.

When you become an RVer, you quickly learn what it means to get a motor home ready for travel. There is an extensive list of prepatory tasks that you go through and the more elaborate the motor home, of course, the longer and more complicated the list becomes. Not to bore you with all the details, but one of the bigger tasks on the list is ensuring the water lines are purged, cleaned and the fresh water tank filled. To do all this though, there is a lot of bending down and standing up work. As you could imagine, this kind of work can be a bit difficult under the circumstances.

Ever since my first relapse, I have had some difficulty with several of my joints, particularly my knees and ankles. Not only are they significantly weaker, but they can at times swell, ache and even downright hurt. Another interesting development since my relapse has been the fact that many of my joints and particularly my knees now squeak. The squeak is accompanied by a sandpaper-like noise that sounds a bit like construction paper tearing. I know that some will say this is nothing more than the cartilage or soft tissue that has worn down in my knees. However true that may be, nothing was squeaking or hurting before the relapse.

This too has become a very distinct memory of my motor home experience as well…right alongside the table and numb back. It can be so quiet outside sometimes when I bend down to either hook up the water line or fill the tank and maybe it's the large surface area of the motor home or something else, but when I stand up from bending down next to the motor home, the noisy knee response is amplified. I would imagine if someone else were standing beside me, they might hear it as well.

While we have made so many great memories on our motor home trips, I don't want to distract from all the good that has come out of it. It does go to show that even the every day, mundane things we would do on any given day can have a significant impact on a person when they have a disease such as MS. And I make this comment realizing that I sit here today a highly-functioning MS patient in the scheme of things. How much harder it most certainly is for those MS patients who have it worse off than I do.

Chapter 25: My Parents

I'm a decade into being a parent myself and there are two truths to parenting (at least that stand way out) that I know to be fact. One, your kids will disproportionately repay you for the things you did yourself as a child. And second, no matter how much you tried growing up to not become your parents, the more and more it seems to be a reality that you will likely turn out to be like your parents.

I have many memories of my mom and dad. Many of these memories are good with a scattering of memories of the not-so-good teenager growing to an adult. But as I matured and got out on my own and then eventually got married, I realized that I had an untapped respect for my parents that grew into a very different understanding of what they did, when they did it and why. I guess the saying is true that you can't know how it really goes until you wear the shoes yourself. And so it has been for me.

I worry myself about the things in life you can't control with kids…their health, their friends, and of course their growing up.

But aside from the normal worries, I haven't had to deal with much in the way of true fear for my kids. Whether it was fear of them getting hurt or being sick, I have not had to experience it, and I thank God every day for that fact. Aside from a rather serious car accident with my mom when I was in high school and the fact that I was very sick as a baby and hospitalized, I don't recall any other events or times in particular that would have created true fear for my parents either.

I remember being a little nervous when I decided to tell my folks about my diagnosis with MS. It was actually before I was officially diagnosed but after we knew something wasn't right and the doctors had prepared us for what was likely to be the diagnosis. I didn't want to wait too long and have them get upset for me not saying anything but didn't want to worry them all the same. It was mostly a matter of appropriately timing things as I was certain I wanted to tell them in person. Delivering the message of my diagnosis was not easy, but they seemed to take the news of my MS well under the circumstances. I'm sure some of it was wishing the best would come of it...and part of it was just the shock of what could be. In any event, they handled it as strong parents would and that ultimately made it so much easier for me to tell them.

I'm glad they have strong friends and family around them as they don't live close to us. We certainly get to visit on the large, regular holidays, but I wish now more than ever we were closer. I imagine it is hard to cope with a situation like this and at the same time there is that helpless feeling of being a parent when you know there really isn't much you can do for your kids to make it better. That is the feeling I fear the most and cannot imagine what it would be like.

But like most things in life, strong people find a way to not only make it through tough situations but find a way to make the most of tough situations. My parents are helping me get through this in a way that can only be accomplished from the role they play of being my mom and dad. This is one of the biggest reasons I love and admire them. It is not for what they physically give me as it may have been when I was young, but rather for the what, how, and when they continue to show me what it means to be a parent.

Chapter 26: Every Step I Take

I have struggled in the recent weeks with a hitch in my step...so to say. This summer has been unbearably hot with temperatures most days in the high 90's. Some days have even been well into the 100's, and then add the high humidity to the mix, and the heat index has ended up well over 110 degrees. I thank God and my work that I have a comfortable job in an air-conditioned environment, and I certainly feel for all those that have to work outside in such conditions. It is literally intolerable.

The hitch that I refer to has been a developing symptom over time, but given the heat...as well as the humidity...the symptom has become extremely exacerbated. Remember what I indicated in an earlier section about body temperature. The higher it gets, the more prevalent symptoms become. And so it has been with several symptoms I have struggled with over the summer. Many of the symptoms are not new, but the difficulty I have walking is.

It seems to all have to do with my right leg. My brain tells my legs to walk without me even really thinking about it, but for some reason my right leg won't lift my foot up all the way so it tends to drag somewhat on the ground. In addition to the drag, my foot turns in a bit, likely because of the physical weight of lifting it. From the drag comes the invariable catching on carpet or an irregular walkway and I am suddenly very unsteady. Add to this an imperfect sense of balance, and I have the ingredients for a good fall.

I haven't actually taken a tumble yet, but I can see how it will likely happen. To be somewhat careful, I tend to walk near the walls in hallways to be "ready" to catch myself. I'm sure I look ridiculous, but probably not as ridiculous as tripping on the carpet in the middle of the hallway and ending up with road rash on my chin. Point being, I think a great deal more about the simple stuff like walking. I am much more thoughtful in my stride and yes it reminds me...really grounds me...in my MS.

Understand, I am thankful for the fact that I can walk so well. I sat in the doctor's office today and watched two different people with walking handicaps related to MS. One of them took nearly an entire minute to get up out of his chair and get his crutches under them. The other one was signing in and literally turned 180 degrees, caught her foot on something, and fell right down in the middle of the floor. Another man close to her stood up and offered her assistance, which she politely refused. I heard her say to him..."This happens all the time. I'm ok. Thank you though." And she got up on her own with a slight smile on her face. Not that I want her disability, but I can tell you, I want her ability. Her ability to suck it up, keep her dignity, get up and go on was absolutely impressive.

I won't be wearing a pedometer any time soon, but I do count my steps. More like I count on my steps in a most different way today than I did before MS. I simply need to get beyond the embarrassment factor and look at it from a perspective of becoming enabled, but not in the sense to not fall down. Falling down happens to everyone whether they have MS or not. Rather, enabled in my mind

means to get up.

Chapter 27: My In-Laws

My wife's parents have always been giving to both of us and have always done a great job of being grandparents to our kids. They are extremely grounded in their ways and have life's priorities in the right order. They aren't burdened by trying to be something they were not intended to be, which is something so many of us get hung up with thinking we have to do...including myself.

Over the years, I have truly come to count on my in-laws as my second family. This doesn't take away from anything my natural parents have done for me in any way. It is merely recognition that I am extremely fortunate to have yet another set of caring, parental heroes to look up to.

I remember years ago before my wife's remaining grandmother passed of her telling how her parents helped with caring for others in the family. Her mom and dad both took full charge and care for their parents. Bathing, feeding, tending and everything else in between went with the territory. They even ended up building on an apartment to their existing home to accommodate an independent yet "ready to be watched" elder. The dedication and commitment this must take cannot really even be put into words.

When it has come to our own family needs, they too have been more than giving to be here for us. Whether spending time with their grandkids or watching the house and family while my wife and I take a little time to ourselves, my in-laws have given freely and without any question. When they learned I had MS, they simply asked how they could help.

It would be utterly amazing to think of a world with more people in it like my in-laws. Thinking of all the good that could and would come from such a thought is overwhelming. Looking back I wish I had more of their qualities in the way I offered help to others. I guess it is never too late though to start. They have had their health issues…their aches and pains…and yet they continue to offer and give freely.

In a big way they inspire me to get my head out of the haze. Their story that I tell myself over and over again reminds me of a better way to think and feel. To be centered in who I am and what I can do and to know that as long as I give it all I have, then the picture is complete. Know the importance of family and never take anything you are given for granted. Be thankful for what you are and have to offer the world. These are the things their actions have taught me.

To look back on the impact they have had on my life since being with their daughter, I won't refer to them as in-laws anymore…they are my other parents.

Chapter 28: Character

In my career in healthcare, I get the chance to do a lot of exciting things. When you consider all the turmoil around healthcare in this country, it is particularly exciting. It is of significant importance to me to know that what I get up to do every day counts. I am a person who wants to see a substantive result that I can say I helped bring about. If my work included only the mundane and unessential aspects of a business or industry, I would not be happy at all. Working with projects of substance and people are important.

What adds such a key ingredient in my work life success and is so often overlooked particularly as a successful trait is the notion of character. I bring this attribute up because there are different "types" of character…all of which contribute, count and speak volumes about a person. With an introspective look while having a disease such as MS, you weigh your own traits very carefully…and if you are being honest with yourself…accurately.

Character means many different things to many different people, but it seems best defined at certain times. I have been around coworkers over the years that I assumed had great character, but looking back over my interactions with them, it was usually involving times of easiness or simple projects. When things got tough, they became a completely different person and not for the better. Character in my opinion can be best described by imagining a grid. On one axis is measured the severity of a situation. On the other axis is the ability to do what is right.

When things are easy, it isn't all that difficult to do what is right. Not to say that some people won't do what is right even then, but you get the picture. As the situation becomes more difficult, the pressure to do what is right becomes increasingly more difficult. This is where character is truly measured. How much harder is it to do the right thing when you know people may be upset or it costs you much more than you would have ever expected...in the most extreme of situations, it could cost you everything.

I am happy with what I believe has been my character trait regarding others. I'm not declaring that I perfectly respond with the right thing all the time or that I do not do wrong. But all in all I believe that I try and succeed in doing what is right even in the wake of difficulty. I would hope that my family, friends and coworkers would say the same. Where I know I have fallen significantly short is my inner character towards myself. This is the character that only affects me regardless of a decision. The benefit or demise completely resides with me. If I don't take care of myself and I eat fast food every day, it will have a significant impact on my health. Now the act of eating right itself is not inner character, but the persistent choice to eat what is right in the wake of passing a burger joint every day is.

I know that my situation with MS is hard. Add to that fact the reality that I am not getting any younger and it is doubly hard. But am I doing everything I need to do? Am I sacrificing and making tough decisions across the board when it comes to my MS? Do I get active and start to contribute to a cure? Do I ever accept any of the handicaps this disease dishes out? As the severity of the situation increases, the decision to do the right thing is staring me stone cold right in the face.

Chapter 29: The Team Concept

The greatest feelings of pride I have ever had have always been associated with a sense of being a part of a team. Whether it was as I remember being young and winning a Little League Championship or the accomplishments I realize today with my team at work, the idea of a team and what a team can do surpasses all the things the same team working as individuals could ever realize. If only I could find a way to get my team to work on the challenge of MS…we would win for certain.

I say this selfishly of course, but the essence of what a successful team can accomplish is almost limitless. I like to say to my teammates today at work…there are certainly some of us who could and some of us who could not accomplish many of the things we take on today as individuals, but there seems almost nothing that we could not accomplish if we all pull together and work together. With the effect of MS on my personal and professional life, I have come to rely to an even greater extent on my team.

I have never been afraid of surrounding myself with people who are quite frankly better than I am. Some leaders are content with having followers who are always "less" than they are. It is a false sense of security to know that you are somehow always better than anyone else on your team. To measure things this way almost always distracts from the real potential an uninhibited team can generate. It can also rob the individuals on a team of what they believe they can truly offer and the cascading effect of this is not only demoralizing but spirit-breaking as well.

The team accepts challenges that would individually be next to impossible to take on. I trust my teammates to look out for each other, to cover all the bases and to catch anything that comes our way. We learn and grow and become better together. When we achieve something triumphant, we celebrate together. When we experience something difficult, we rally, learn and grow.

I am trying to find how the team concept fits in with my personal fight against MS. On the one hand I have a great team...my family…to help me through this. I also have a great team at work that understands and steps up to take on tasks and projects when I am unable. But I know there is more that a team could do rather than just me on my own. I sense this starts by getting more involved. To spark a fire that could contribute to helping others who fight this battle would be a powerful team effort. Maybe in a way writing this book is my start.

Chapter 30: Perspective

This is one of those areas that quite frankly has always been difficult for me to grasp. To put myself in someone else's shoes and realize, feel and experience things from their side. Oh sure, I have said on many occasions that I understand someone's position, even that I sympathize or empathize with their dilemma, but no matter how old or mature I become, I never really get this one down.

I think it may be this way for a lot of people. Then again, how easy is it really to do? I can't really be in someone else's shoes...I'm in my shoes. To even think that all the events that may have led up to a seemingly bad decision or what I may view as a "dumb" choice are not even mine to speak about. In the end, all I see is the result, and if we all knew the result before we did certain things, we would likely know precisely what we should do to get a better result by doing it a different way, or making a different decision than we actually did.

But now move to other aspects of life where things happen to us and we have no input or control over them. We don't make the wrong choice…we don't make a choice at all. We have to play a bad hand that was merely dealt our way. While I know it is easier for me to at least understand a situation such as this for someone, it is still just as hard to know their perspective. I have certainly come to at least know how rotten this is for anyone in this situation. It isn't fair. It isn't warranted. It makes the person question so much in and about their own life.

It has come down to such primary reasoning for my own situation with MS. Did I do something to deserve this? Did I not do something to deserve this? Why did this happen to me? I'm a pretty good person. I know I haven't been perfect but this can't be happening to me. These are all aspects of the lonely side of perspective when you have to spend time thinking about your own self. There isn't another person that I can pretend to wear their shoes. When I look down they are my shoes that I wear.

I have struggled for over a year trying to keep things in perspective and another year prior trying to figure out my perspective…and I still know that I don't have it down. Maybe the hardest part with perspective is knowing that it is never static…it will always change. Just as my life with MS will undoubtedly be different in three years or five years, so will my perspective on my life with MS. The fact that there isn't a "right" perspective that I can always reference back to or rely on for the rest of my life makes it very scary.

It is funny how our minds work. We spend so much time thinking about the things we want to do with our lives and comparatively how we stack up against others that we literally lose sight of ourselves. We lose our true perspective and the only way we can relate from then on is by trying to put ourselves in other people's situations and spinning how we would have done things differently. For being such a smart species, we sure can sometimes get it all wrong. Maybe it takes events such as getting MS to get us back to what is really important…what is truly in perspective.

I know for me that I am focusing on things much differently now. I will also admit that I have been forced to do it because of my MS. Whatever the reason, I have a different outlook on things. I know I need to take these life lessons and be perceptive in an open and honest way. There isn't anyone else to ask to step into my shoes and see it from my eyes. Perspective is ultimately rooted in reality whether we like it or not. Whether I choose to realize this or not can either help or hurt me.

I firmly believe that part of the journey I must travel for myself is to someday be entirely able to never lose my life's perspective. To not let the mundane or passing time get the better of me and forget where it is I am and how I got there. If having MS helps me with this, then in a way there is certainly some good that will come of this disease. Knowing that this in and of itself is such an awkward and profound logic to follow is evidence enough for us to all try the same.

Chapter 31: My Boss

You might be thinking why someone would write a section in a book about MS on their boss. What does this have to do with anything? Truth is my boss is one of the individuals who has helped me get to a better place with my disease. No, he has not been actively involved in my disease management. He has not held my hand through the multitude of tests. And no, he has not taken care of my medical bills. But what he has done is just as important and thoughtful.

I have known him for many years, but he has only been my boss for the past four. We are very similar in many ways, but his leadership and experience far surpass my own current skill set. His commitment to his work, the perfect conclusion he strives to achieve, and his determination to make a difference are in lock step with my own work ethic. He is a man of his word, and I am proud to call him a friend and teammate.

His work history is humble. He earned everything he has gotten through his effort and skill. And now he is the COO of our company. But even in the wake of his success, he has been one of the most understanding individuals throughout this entire ordeal for me. He has always been there and is ever persistent in his support.

Not too long ago, he himself ran into a rather significant health issue. Over the years, he has struggled with a degenerative back disorder and about four months ago aggravated it to the point of daily impact on his life. It is a painful disorder and has consumed him mentally and physically. Throughout his own ordeal he has practiced what he has preached to me for the past year. Most if not all of the positive qualities I speak about in this book he shows through his own thoughts, responses and actions. He has shown me through his own personal situation how best to direct my own actions towards my MS.

For most people, they never really get to know the other side of their leaders, the personal, exposed and frail side. Most only know what they see at work or in meetings. They only see what the leader wants them to see. But leaders are only human like the rest of us. Bad things happen to them and their families just like anyone else. When a leader reaches out as my boss has to me, it means even more because they are showing and accepting of the vulnerabilities that can afflict any of us.

It wasn't easy sharing my story with him, not so much from how he would react but more to the point of me telling him of this weakness I now had. I did not want him to think any less of me and here I was trying to explain how this disease was taking things away from me. MS could make me less of a contributor, less of a man, and yes, less of a leader. I was scared that he would see me for what MS was doing to me. But he didn't. He helped me hold my head high. I was relieved to know he was behind me by standing with me.

He will soon undergo surgery to help with his back, and I suspect that in the aftermath he will continue to persevere with the same energy and effectiveness he has always possessed. That too will help me with what I must undergo. Although my journey may end up taking me a bit longer down the road of recovery, I am extremely grateful for what he has given me. His understanding and pure acceptance while not assuming me to be less than I was before I told him about my MS is a testament to who he really is. I have always known him to be a sincere person, but his character and leadership has been validated through his own struggle and how he has encouraged me through mine.

Part Two: Understanding to Accepting

There really is no magical moment or "A-ha" to cross over to total understanding. As you can probably tell from the topics in Part One understanding is itself similar to MS in that it is progressive. You come to understand the disease more and more. You come to understand yourself more and more. You come to understand how both coexist more and more. But there is a point at which you have enough understanding that you can begin to move toward acceptance. It is not a definitive line you cross but rather a shaded area. One day you are more on one side of the shaded area, and at some point in the future, you are more on the other side.

There is a crossover though, and I believe you will know when you are there. It was that way for me, and after speaking with my doctor who has seen hundreds if not possibly thousands of MS patients over his career, I would think he too would agree. Sometimes your own sense of understanding and ultimate acceptance is rooted in the fact that others around you seem to be moving down this path as well. Maybe it's your family or friends. Maybe it's a coworker or your church. The people around you that show you support will be a catalyst to your own acceptance of this disease.

A great analogy that you can draw a parallel on is the path of a professional athlete. While there are certainly athletes throughout history that would claim to have made it on their own, most would probably not only give credit to their own individual effort but also the effort of many people around them. They too would point to their families, coaches, trainers, doctors, teammates and even fans. Without the efforts and attention from these other individuals who have understood, aided, trained, taught, encouraged, supported, coached and believed, these athletes would not be the shadow of what they were ultimately able to achieve.

Yet whatever the effort given by others, those with this disease have to be willing to give even more. To break through simply understanding to a state of pure acceptance is the foundation to winning the battle against MS. It is ultimately here that you draw the

power to clear the hurdles MS will place in front of you. And there

will be hurdles. At times when you are hurting or painfully reminded

in some way that you have this disease, you can always draw upon the

safety of your acceptance to bring you back to a grounded state. And

it is here that you will find the spark…that inner strength to keep

things in perspective and discover how to win.

Chapter 32: Patience

This is a quality I assure you I do not have in sufficient quantities. I have always been a rather impatient person when it comes to most everything. From looking at a list full of tasks I know I have to get done all the way to what I expect from the world around me, if you expect me to get through it with a high degree of patience, it becomes ten times harder. If something is broke, I want to fix it. I don't want to wait patiently for someone else to do it.

I remember going through the medical trials and tribulations of finding out what was wrong which ultimately led to my diagnosis with MS. It was frustrating. It was not that people weren't trying to figure it out, but the fact that the answer wasn't so simple to find naturally caused me to kick in my profound sense of impatience. Why was this taking so long? Can't someone see what is going on under a microscope and just tell me what it is? There was no logical way in my speed-possessed mind to figure things out, and this ultimately would manifest into a sense of near desperation to get an answer.

I'm sure you have heard the saying that "patience is a virtue". At some point in my early struggle to grasp hold of something that would make this easier, I remember thinking of my grandfather. My dad's dad was a great man. He was a German descendant who was very skilled with his hands. He owned a dry cleaning store, was a tailor as well as a master woodworker. He made a living for his family from these skills. I remember being young and examining some of the things he had made. They were so precise and perfectly crafted. His meticulous effort would leave most people in awe. It certainly did me.

He was always so patient with me. I was the young grandson always moving and never sitting still. He could always find a way to hold my attention. His actions kept me focused. It almost seemed like it was effortless for him. The more I thought about him the more I attributed his success not only in dealing with a high-strung grandson but in all that he was able to accomplish in life to the virtue of patience. Later in his life I recall, a tremor-like trait he had developed that was rather evident in his hands. It was not related to anything in particular…likely just from getting older.

I would watch him as he would attempt to do things and was amazed at how calm and patient he would be with himself. I even remember my dad telling me of how hard it would be for him to do something like thread a needle, but he was able to master it even with an unsteady hand. He would grab the thread in one hand and the other would hold the needle. With both hands shaking, he would move them closer together. To the observer you would think it was going to take a while. There was no way he is going to get that needle threaded. But he did. And it didn't take him several attempts; it didn't even take him more than one. Time and time again, he would hit the needle's eye flawlessly in the wake of that perpetual shake.

This one simple act summed up how my grandfather held true to the virtue of patience. The thought of this one simple act still moves me to this day. In all the turmoil that I can create in my own mind by not having patience, I can hold on to this one thought and somehow it makes it better. I know what he was able to accomplish and maintain through patience can be a buoy of inspiration to me. It is my refuge.

Always reach for something that gives you the same.

Chapter 33: Self Reliance

I recall reading Ralph Waldo Emerson in high school and an essay he wrote on self reliance. It was both eloquent and profound, but what I recall the essay surmised in the end was that a true sense of living at peace comes only from one place...ourselves. Of course reading it when I was sixteen or seventeen, I am pretty sure that statement would have sounded rather corny. In our society today, we come so quickly and easily to rely on so many external factors at play. Technology provides for conveniences never thought of twenty or even ten years ago. Society pushes us in one direction or another, and we ebb and flow to a tune created not from ourselves.

As the years roll by in our lives, more and more enters to influence how we view not only ourselves but our outlook on life. The culmination of the things in our lives and the events of our lives shape and mold not only our physical self but our mental outlook on practically all things. For many of us and certainly in my case, we can end up further and further from our true self. We no longer view ourselves as a source of sustainability or happiness, but turn to the world and all that is in it to fill us.

Self reliance was a much closer concept people could grasp long ago. Life depended on it. The ability for an individual or family to truly make a living by what they literally did, how they thought, the decisions they made, and the ideas they acted on were in many ways essential. Life wasn't harder, but living certainly was. But people of that time didn't worry so much about the quantity of time they spent on this earth. It was more a mission to ensure quality of time. Living a better, more robust life was the primary focus, and the sustainability of this concept was rooted in one's ability to count on one's self.

While today we enjoy so many unthinkable conveniences in life compared to people a century ago, that same mission to ensure quality of time still lies within each of us. The sad thing for most today is realizing this mission is as elusive as it was then…maybe even more so. I know this sounds a bit ironic given everything we think we have available to us compared to those of long ago, but it points to an inner need that slips silently away over time.

This notion of self reliance that I am speaking of is not necessarily the idea of self sustainability. My point is not to say you have to find a way to do everything on your own...grow your own vegetables, build your own house, make your own living. Rather the idea of self reliance is a state of mind to know that you can count on yourself...believe in yourself...find that inner peace. And what is inner peace? I believe this will be different for everyone. The state of being at peace with yourself can be compared to your appetite. One person might be satisfied with a small meal...another person may require larger portions.

The mission though is ultimately the same. Being comfortable and confident in how you think and feel about yourself, knowing how you can and will get something accomplished, and then making it happen are the anchors of self reliance referred to here. I am amazed at how so many MS patients have an obvious sense of self reliance.

What stands in their way is tackled by the instinctive trait they have nurtured through relying on their own self. I believe you can see this same trait in so many people that cope with a life-changing illness. To the casual observer, they read about people such as this and think what this person has done is amazing. How possibly could someone with such a debilitating challenge do it? To the one they are asking this question, the answer is actually quite simple; it was done because they have developed a natural trust with themselves to know they can do it.

I think for me the very point at which I knew I had accepted MS in my life was the exact point at which I was at peace with it. It was the point I knew I had the inner confidence to embrace my situation and own it as mine. Even though I don't know throughout the rest of my life all the things I will have to call upon to deal with MS, I do know that I can count on myself to face it. I trust the reliance I have placed on myself to be there for that challenge. The world in all it has to offer can only push from the outside. The domain you possess as your true self pushes from inside you out onto the world.

Self reliance is a big part of your personal push. In all that remains uncertain in this world today as it did a century ago, I know you can find true peace by believing in what you can do for yourself.

Chapter 34: Determination

If there was a short list of qualities that I have always admired in a person regardless of our differences, one in particular would be the person that possesses sheer determination. Most of the experiences I remember were being around people that were not destined to do what they were attempting. Determination isn't really needed when things come easy. In fact, it is the individual that stretches for things they cannot do as they dig deep to find inside themselves what originally was not there, and then create something from what seemed to be nothing.

Determination is first tested by one's ability to sustain a situation. When you meet someone who has been diligent and consistent in dealing with a situation…they haven't taken the easy way out by giving up or making excuses as to why they were not able to get to their desired result, more times than not you can point to their ability to remain determined as a major key to their success.

Determination is not a beginning or an end; it is cohesiveness. It acts more like the stickiness that keeps things together.

I can remember back over my life and really only find a few times that I have truly engaged my sense of determination...I mean the kind of determination that creates a different you. I am determined to be a great husband and father to my wife and kids. I have the determination to be the best I can at my career. I am determined to be a good son and help my parents when they need me. Situations such as this we all will likely experience. When the opportunity presents itself for me to be more than I am at that particular time, I know that what is really being tested is my determination.

I can honestly say I have not ever had to possess any level of determination to something that may take up the rest of my life. To think of MS this way makes it feel like a daunting and lifelong task with an unknown future. But like so many things in life, determination is a choice. I can choose to maintain a sense of determination to fight this disease and stay true to myself or I can find another reason to allow my determination to give way to something else…like self-pity or settling for a loss. I don't know about you, but while I don't like to lose, I believe I would like it even less if I lose because I did not give myself the chance.

Being determined is a daily choice, and it is not easy; I know. It is not something you inherit. Days will turn into weeks, weeks to months and months to years. Determination must be nurtured to keep pace with the situation. Yet I know that if I stay focused; remain patient and self reliant, I can find determination to come easier. Determination fosters hope and hope fosters health. Investing in myself in this way will give me the edge that I need. Carrying determination in my MS tool belt and choosing to use it every day will bring about a result that would not have been there without it.

Chapter 35: Watch the Rain

Have you ever had the fortune of watching a rain shower while it is sunny? It is hypnotic to watch the sun almost light up each individual rain drop as it falls. As more and more of them fall from the sky, no two rain drops will travel the same path or land in exactly the same place. The randomness of it literally looks uniform in the end. Such a small thing in and of itself ends up covering virtually everything in its path. The ground gets blanketed by it, but it all started with a single rain drop. If you take this to a global level in the same thought, the earth ends up in its entirety, albeit at a different frequency, getting covered by rain. Think of how many drops it must take to make this ultimately happen. And yet it does. Through the randomness of weather patterns and mixed precipitation, the result is a complete blanketing of the globe.

I'm sure scientists have a technical name for this, but in my simple mind it is just an awesome thing when I think about it. Years ago I probably would have never even taken the time to stop and think about something so seemingly ridiculous. But I sure think of these things now. I try to apply thoughts such as this to my own life to learn a little something from them. There is such a sense of completeness and perfectness in so many things we come in contact with in life if you just take the time to realize it.

Life feels so different with MS. Sometimes it feels hard, but at other times it can feel refreshing. I am looking at so many things from a different perspective and shame on me that it took a disease like MS to make me see it. But no matter the reason, my outlook is different and that I believe is a great thing. As I go through life, I know I will get rained on, just as I did before MS. What falls on me isn't really the point, but how I choose to take it and what I make of it is.

For me it is rooted in my faith. For someone else it may be something else. But I believe that the things that happen in our lives happen for a reason. Just as we generally overlook the rain, we have a tendency to overlook most things that fall on our lives. We generally only start looking closer at them when they are things we do not want to fall on us. I have learned to not let this be the case. I think about my MS every day, but I also think about so many other things that cover me and rain on me day in and day out too. I look to make sense of things more often and learn from them. I look not only to understand them but to also accept them. What would life really be like without the rain? I say it wouldn't be much of a life at all.

Chapter 36: Carpe Diem

I recall a high school English teacher that was big on this particular saying. She would even write it on the board throughout the year for different reasons, but it always read the same...Carpe Diem. "Seize the day" she would say to our class of inattentive students. Of course, when you are fifteen or sixteen, you are only concerned with driving, snowboarding, girls and your friends. How much more could I have seized the day than that? I guess it is one of those sayings that really only sinks in with time and life experiences. As time passes, the statement means even more.

I see so many people, including myself, that believe in seizing the day, but we have no intention of getting started on it until tomorrow. Why is that? Lob it right up there with other things that we completely realize and even believe are things we should be doing today, but we find every reason in the book to procrastinate doing any of them. How consistently we remain in the same rut of life taking the easy way down the road, we really don't seize any of our days; we just

141

casually cruise through them. I know that I think about days like this now with intense disappointment in myself. And yes, it took MS to bring me to this.

In all my idleness I look today at a few lucky people out there who have chosen to step on the throttle and live. They do not just do it in a reckless manner but are smart and deliberate to get the most out of everything they put effort into doing. My parents are pretty good at it, but even they seemed to save the time to do it for their retirement. A saying that has stuck with me for many years goes like this, "You live your life only once, but if you live right; once is enough." This is not only a profoundly accurate statement for anyone, but is also an absolute depiction of seizing not just the day but every day.

My goal is to wake up with energy and go to bed tired. In between, I want to make the most of every minute I have. For me it isn't so much about using this time to collect the trophies in life but more about what I can give back. With the talents I have even though they may be or become inhibited by MS over time, I can still give in a creative and productive way. There will always be someone else out there in the world that has it worse off than me so making excuses or feeling sorry for myself does nothing. To put it quite simply, it robs me of seizing the day.

I believe that seizing any day begins with realizing it is better to give than to get. It involves being respectful of our time and other's time. It is intimately attached to effort and attempt no matter how many times we may fail. Think of how great we, our communities, even our country could be if we treated every day this way. Carpe diem did not only apply to people of the past, it applies to all of us today and to our futures. Seizing the day is a state of mind that completely satisfies. It can unlock potential and open our eyes.

I know I need to wake up every day choosing things differently than I have in the past. In a way writing this book is evidence for me that I am at least starting to make better decisions toward truly seizing my days. Quite frankly it feels good. The memories I have of days like this are more vivid, colorful and satisfying. When you are able to

143

seize just one day, it becomes addictive. Of all the things we are told

about addictions, this one wouldn't be that bad at all for any of us to

have.

Chapter 37: Choices to Make

Try explaining the concept of choices to a six year old. They grasp the concept vaguely when you are talking about choosing between one type of candy versus another; but put it in a higher realm like good and bad choices in life, and they get lost quickly. And why wouldn't they, their youthful situations do not call for significant choices just yet. My two older kids are beginning to feel the essence of choice. My wife and I try to give them choices and help them to understand the consequences of their decisions. We certainly do not let them get into trouble with their decisions, but we believe making choices today on simple situations or circumstances are great life lessons.

I remember a conversation I had with my twins recently as I was attempting to explain to them that so much of what we will face in our lives involves making choices. Sometimes we come from very different backgrounds and lessons in life. Some have been abused or neglected. Some have been given virtually everything to meet every need. Nevertheless, we arrive at different places not only because of our past but because of the choices we make along the way. Some choices are harder to arrive at than others. As well it may take one person longer, or they may need to take a different path to get to the same place. In any case, our decisions about what lies ahead in our path either gets us through it, around it, or stopped by it.

An ironic thought that came to mind after talking with my kids about this subject was that of my own situation. Sickness is certainly not something most of us choose. While there are some illnesses such as lung cancer that could have been prevented by choosing not to smoke in some cases, there are other illnesses that arrive in our lives complete without choice. So it has been in my case with MS. The best I can tell and as supported by most in the medical profession, maybe it was a viral infection when I was young, or a deficiency in vitamin D, maybe it has been some combination of chemicals I was exposed to or some other neurological anomaly, whatever the cause, it was not something I chose and yet the consequence was MS.

The fact that MS has happened in my life and as to the why it happened, I will leave to the doctors to figure out. What is of greater importance are the choices I make from this point forward about it. I can choose to give up or step up. I can feel sorry for myself or feel blessed for everything that makes my life worth living. Bottom line, the choice is mine. When I arrived at that place of understanding MS as a part of my life and moved into the world of accepting my MS, the choices surrounding me did get easier. In fact, the choices I make now seem to have much higher stakes. Then again, most choices are as you mature and move on in your life.

Thinking back on the conversation I had with my kids, I guess I was not only speaking to them, but I was speaking to myself as well. I owe it to myself and to my family and friends to make the best choices I can. It doesn't matter that I have MS; it doesn't matter that MS is yet another factor that plays into the decisions I must make. What matters is that I still have a choice how to live, and MS did not take that choice away from me.

Chapter 38: Maintain a Healthy Mind

If you think about it, to an MS patient having a healthy mind is a bit of an oxymoron. Maybe the technical oxymoron would be having a healthy brain, but you get my drift. As much as MS physically attacks the gray matter, it doesn't mean that you cannot maintain a healthy mind. While this can certainly apply to all of us, it is an especially important point to an MS patient. To think positive is paramount to your overall health. It gives you the edge to realize your potential, and this point is a key element to moving from accepting the disease to ultimately beating it.

Have you ever seen a cancer patient that has gone through months or maybe even years of grueling hardships and still smile about it? To the untrained eye it would appear this person may be in absolute denial, but to the astute observer they will see much more. They will see a person who has maintained a flawless affinity to keep their mind healthy and happy. I get glimpses of this myself from time to time. I know I could easily slip away into a negative frame of mind, but I find myself looking at the brighter side…seeing the good in a situation…reaching out for a better end to the story. Admittedly I realize I am not perfect nor will I ever be. Yet more and more I try to keep a healthy frame of mind regarding my MS and while this isn't always the easiest path to take, it almost always ends up being the most rewarding.

I seem to feel so much better in the aftermath if I know I tried to do something with a positive and healthy frame of mind. For some reason, even if I don't succeed in what I set out to do or accomplish, the memories of the attempt or effort are so much richer and clearer knowing that I tried with the right frame of mind. Even when I do fail, a healthy frame of mind can set me up to succeed the next time. Can you imagine what the world would be like if all of our efforts were always attempted with a positive and healthy frame of mind? This very thought captures the essence of my desire.

A big part of successfully living with MS is not only found in moving from a complete sense of understanding into accepting…it is moving through both the right way. Someone may come to understand their MS but for all the wrong reasons. They may come to resent the disease…they may even hate it. The negative, unhealthy energy that this generates will only prove to set in motion an unfortunate and destructive state of acceptance. Even though MS has not been shown to shorten a person's life, however debilitated they may become, it seems to me the greater debilitating result would be if understanding and acceptance were based on hatred and resentment towards the disease.

To truly realize what you are ultimately capable of begins and ends with thinking and seeing yourself doing the very thing you intended to accomplish. MS will try to distract you from this as will other hurdles in life. Don't let it. The richness of a healthy mind-based effort can create a purity of clear vision and spirit. This is where you can begin to win. This is the beginning to where all things are possible.

Chapter 39: Perseverance

How many times have we all been tested? In life...in our work...even in our families, we have all seen a point at one time or another when we desperately want to just say "I give". Giving up is a very natural conclusion to many challenges and hardships that we have or may face. In fact, if you look across many different species, including humans, giving up is a survival instinct. It is a way to safely secure our future or in the very least our tomorrow.

If you ever want to witness this point in the purest sense, read about how a wolf pack functions. When two strong-willed wolves clash, the race for dominance commences. The build up to the episode could take weeks or months, but in the end it generally comes down to a climactic event. In the heat of battle, one wolf will take a commanding advantage and at some point the other wolf will yield...or give up. Order is restored and the hierarchy is clear. The defeated wolf knows where they stand, but has survived to fulfill a lesser role in the pack.

In much the same way as wolves in a pack, there are numerous clashes that I know I will likely face with my disease. The position of dominance will ultimately be determined in a similar way. But giving up is taking a position of acceptance that is quite literally unacceptable to me. The notion of acceptance if it means taking a "lesser role in the pack" will simply not do. But I know it will be a hard fight, and I will need something much more than just a solid sense of understanding to claim dominance.

This is where perseverance plays a vital role...and at times even a lead role. The definition of perseverance goes beyond just being determined. It is the idea of being determined consistently...day in and day out. Perseverance does not know the notion of giving up or stopping. It is not wild or uncontrolled. It is deliberate and steady. It is not being perfect, but it is perfecting your effort.

Admittedly I have doubts about how I will persevere against MS. I have days when it would be much easier to give up...survive...and accept a lesser position. If I don't try something, then I won't have to admit defeat. It is another way of giving up but without even attempting. But something rubs me wrong when I think of this as a possible way out. I feel cheap. I feel I have literally cheated myself, my family and friends. For all that I have inside myself and everything so many have invested in me to be the person I am today, this is not a viable road to travel. Perseverance creates the needed medium for me to not act on the easy way out. It doesn't promise victory, but it certainly keeps me on the path.

My acceptance is not just about the reality of MS in my life, but it is also accepting what I believe I am capable of doing about it. To persevere in what I believe I can do makes me a consistent and constant fighter. A boxer, like the wolf, doesn't fight to simply win a round. He doesn't fight to give up in the end. He fights to be victorious. And like the wolf, he goes into the battle knowing that even though at any given minute of the fight he could be down, he perseveres to the next minute and the next so that he can embrace victory. Consistent and constant determination...perseverance to the point of seeing my victory so clearly that all I have to do is accept it…that is what I want to feel.

Chapter 40: Turn Wishing to Hope

I remember when I was younger...much younger...sitting around the formal dining room table. This is the table and room that I was perpetually told not to play in, on or around. It was the room that we only used on special occasions so birthdays were justly included. Someone would say as the candles were about to be blown out, "Make a wish." This was my cue, and I took it seriously. I would close my eyes and bear down hard to make that wish; I really wanted it to come true.

Wishing rarely got me what I really wanted, but every time someone would say those words I would indulge myself to repeat the same exercise practically every time. It is amazing how I have gone through life making wishes. Even as an adult I would say to myself and in my own mind the words would start off "I wish..." Wishing even played a part after I discovered I had MS. I would wish it to go away. I would wish I was normal. I would even wish after seeing another MS patient in the doctor's office to not end up like them.

Like when I was young, wishing hasn't gotten me very far. It is more fantasy than anything. Wishing is blind. It doesn't see you to anything of substance. It can create a short-lived and wildly-opportunistic thought or idea that fizzles out quickly. It gives you nothing to build from or towards.

At some point in my journey from understanding to accepting, maybe through my own maturing with this disease or by the calming effect that understanding seems to bring, I started to turn from wishing to hope. Hope is a very different feeling than wishing. Hope means so much more particularly to a person who genuinely needs it. The feeling itself is contagious and seems to positively spread to others. It can inspire not only the very person in hope but those around them as well.

Turning a wish into a hope means moving an outward request from chance to an earnest expectation. It is a constructive conversion from an inexperienced plea to a mature and meaningful desire. Hope can inspire a person to do something or to realize something that may not have been possible without it. Hope establishes trust not only within one's self but outwardly as well.

I am not wishful for a cure, but I am hopeful for one. Because of this, I know that I will find ways beyond this book to help myself and hopefully others to get there. I am not going to rely on circumstance or chance to be the basis for realizing this; I am going to mindfully hope and have an earnest expectation of myself and others to do all that is necessary to move forward towards a cure, towards a better tomorrow for those in my shoes. Wishing for such a bold result is merely a desperate plea. There are no candles to blow out and even if there were, it would provide nothing after the candles were extinguished. Having MS has taught me to hope for so much more in my life. In fact, I don't even think I will look at another birthday cake the same way.

Chapter 41: Some Days Will Be Tough

Do you ever recall learning about sound waves in school? The wavy line has peaks and troughs and the frequency determines how many of them will be evident over a period of time. Although not a sound wave, you can see a perfect example of this if you look at a heartbeat on an electrocardiogram. The cardiac rhythm or wave moves up and down with every beat of the heart. It is almost visually soothing to see as it is evidence of us being alive.

The life I live with MS parallels this very up and down wave in an almost perfect fashion. For that matter, the ups and downs of anyone's life find rhythm to this same result. But within life's ups and downs, there are also the ups and downs I experience from MS as well. It is almost like an overlay wave to the wave of life. Sometimes it follows similar peaks and valleys as life; sometimes they are off and out of sync. Life in general may be up or riding a peak when an inconvenient setback or trough occurs with MS. As with most things in life, very few events or circumstances happen out of convenience or at least when we want them to.

About a month or so ago, we took our two boys to the 100-year anniversary Boy Scout Jamboree. It was mid fall and we were expecting it to be relatively cool. In addition, we were not aware when we arrived how spread out the event was and how it would require extensive walking. I had every intention of hanging tough through the event and given different circumstances probably could have done just that. But as it turned out, the temperature reached into the 90's and the walk just from where we parked to the main part of the events was over a mile. I barely got to where we were going, and I knew I wouldn't make the day. By lunchtime, I had to go back to the truck and spend the remainder of the day resting in an air conditioned vehicle. I not only felt like I had let my kids and family down…I had let myself down. The reality of the situation was my MS rhythm ended up out of sync from the rhythm of life.

I have learned to listen to my body more attentively and watch for changes in my "MS wave". I have to. To not pay attention to what this wave is doing, what is going on with my MS peaks and valleys, can be detrimental. To be more astutely aware of this wave though can also cause me to read into things more and lose some of the joy when things are going well. Why? If I realize that I am in a peak, I presume the wave will begin to move downward towards a trough. I start to think about the downward trend instead of enjoying the high of the wave. In the same way I could be in a valley and "expect" to soon be moving to a peak. The expectation of this can be disappointing when it doesn't seem to happen on my timeline. It can be a tricky mental balance to not over anticipate what weather may be coming my way.

Regardless of how much or how little I anticipate the wave, I do know that it will continue to ebb and flow. At times it will be up and other times it will be down. Part of the acceptance process is grasping this as yet another layer of ups and downs on my already wavy life and riding it no matter where it is. Some days will be great and some days will be tough. MS does make the valleys seem lower, but surprisingly I will admit it can make the peaks feel higher. I know it sounds crazy; but when I feel good, I realize how much I have taken previous peaks for granted. I seem to revel in it more and have a deeper value for the time.

I won't sugarcoat the troughs though, they can be very tough. I have to call upon more mental aptitude to get beyond it. The biggest part of a trough is realizing that there will be more and being astutely aware of how I am feeling and what my body is doing to respond to the MS. As time goes on, I get better and better at it. I am even taking this awareness to a higher level by applying the same principles to my larger life wave.

Most of us through our normal course of life do not take the time to listen or read what our bodies are telling us until it is too late. We eat too much of the things that are bad for us, exercise too little, and overindulge in the conveniences of life only to end up with a catastrophic health event that shocks us into paying more attention to our waves. MS has taught me to not wait until then. Look at the wave now and all the other little waves that intersect my life today. I know not to expect only peaks but am better prepared to move into a trough, through it as well as out of it.

MS will always present a future low spot on the curve. It will always have troughs and valleys. Acceptance fosters preparation rather than anticipation. It creates a venue by which the accepting MS patient can better read and navigate the curve regardless of where they are on the curve. The energy to travel the curve is more productive and like the wave of your own heartbeat, it is much more meaningful and a necessary part of life.

Chapter 42: Inspiration

There are some movies that I have watched in recent years that with the new visual technologies available today seem to turn into awesome spectacles of sound and sight. You can see details and hear things never before imagined on a big screen. It makes it so much easier to really get into the show. And if my imagination takes over, I can find myself caught up in the action imagining what I might be capable of doing. It gets my adrenaline going and makes me feel like I am somehow as big as the actors on the screen.

Now don't get me wrong, I am not going to run out and try to pull off some of the crazy things I may see in a movie, but my point is more to the way the situation makes me feel. To put it simply, it can be inspiring. I like the feeling. It makes me feel more alive and heightens my senses. I have a clearer mind and can dream bigger. Inspiration is healthy particularly for someone with MS. There are so many things that work to drag you down, it is essential to find things that counter this effect.

Inspiration is fuel. It is fuel for the soul, mind, and body. You cannot dredge it up by taking a pill or willing it to happen. It is placed on us like a blanket in a very delicate manner. I heard someone say one time that when you are young you never really can experience inspiration because it never has time to develop. Kids are so energetic that when the "feeling" of inspiration blankets them, it turns into a burst of energy that they immediately act on. As you get older and lose this sense of instant energy, the blanket has time to develop and inspiration takes its place. Energy and inspiration can both result in positive action and maybe even help you realize you can do more than you thought you could.

I believe as I have gotten older, I am truly inspired to a lesser degree. It seems this is the case for most of us. Yet when I am inspired, it seems to be much more meaningful. Since being diagnosed with MS, I tend to be so preoccupied with what the disease is doing to me that I have a tendency to miss when the blanket of inspiration may be upon me. My kids inspire me. My wife inspires me. And yet so many times I can miss it.

Inspiration is certainly something to savor. It seems to add years to your life even if it is only for a brief period of time. Inspiration dares you to do something different. I know with MS I have to do things differently; I have to think things differently. As this disease takes things away, I have to be able to find the energy to counter this effect. Inspiration provides this opportunity.

How much better are we when we do things we are inspired to do? How much more rewarding are results when they come from an inspired action? Life is simply more when it is inspired life.

Chapter 43: Talk to Others with MS

I know I am not the only one with MS. I also know that I do not have it nearly as bad as some …at least at this point in my life. I have been extremely fortunate. I found a great doctor early on in my discovery process which has helped me to get a jump on a regular treatment path. Up until about 25 years ago, there really were no FDA-approved treatment options specifically for MS. It is a younger disease in this regard.

However, there are numerous patients that have been diagnosed with MS long before any treatment options were available. Sure they may be older than I am, but they have a wealth of knowledge from their experiences. And in many cases, their symptoms are much more severe today because they went so long without routine MS treatment during the earlier years of their diagnosis. While it is a bit hard to look into their eyes and not picture myself facing a similar fate, acceptance has helped me to look past their façade and see what lies behind their eyes and into their thoughts, their energy, and their outlook on life.

So many patients with MS have learned to talk to other patients because the disease is so unique to each of us. It is not only interesting to learn what others are dealing with, but important to listen to what they have done about it. No it doesn't mean that what may have worked for them will work for me, yet the information is educational, and learning more helps me to sort through my options.

Many of these patients have found the peace of understanding and acceptance. You can hear it in their voices and see it on their faces. They push through the lows and ride long and hard on the highs. They have truly integrated MS into their lives and not the other way around. Their words exude encouragement for me and show me that they too are conquering their MS through a journey of personal success. They rely on their own efforts, they lean on the help of family and friends, they hold true to their treatment, and they are extremely thoughtful and deliberate in their actions.

Others with MS can help to create a network of support that can be a valuable tool to a newly diagnosed patient. It is almost like a freshman in high school that learns to look up to the role model of an upper classman. Placing yourself in this network will be a certain benefit, but the focus has to be on constructive interaction. Look for other patients who possess the understanding and acceptance that you seek. If someone is constantly talking about the "bad" with their MS, if their words are discouraging and full of resentment, then they are not traveling the right road. They may be early in their journey or not on the right path at all, but it will be obvious if you listen. In contrast, the understanding and accepting patients will truly talk about themselves and how they have integrated MS into their lives. The focus will be on their accomplishments and what they have overcome. You will feel their energy and excitement of how they have been victorious time and time again through all the situations where MS has tried to knock them down. This is the patient that gets it; this is the person to listen to.

It is a great exercise to talk to others with MS and network with them so that you can learn to listen better to yourself. When you hear yourself becoming discouraged, you can relate it back to a similar patient who was talking in the same way. It can help to flip the switch to get you back on the right track. Like you, other proactive patients are also listening in the same way. Learning to make yourself a better person with MS can be a beacon for others that are new to the disease, and the time will certainly present itself when you will be able to share your journey and help someone to reach out for the same success.

Chapter 44: Don't Be Ashamed

I have been so sensitive to how people will perceive me now with MS that it has been very easy to slip into the coma of shame. I have felt shame when other fathers are able to help out with their kid's sports and I can't. I have felt shame when I couldn't find a way to get back into woodworking. I even see shame creeping into my thoughts about what MS may do to me in the future to prevent me from being the man I know I will need to be.

Being ashamed is a very vulnerable feeling. It is defined as a painful emotion resulting from an awareness of inadequacy or guilt. Shame is like a cancer. It can spread quickly and move through every fiber of your existence. It can pounce on your conscience and occupy so much of your mind and effort; it is poisonous.

I have struggled so intently with measuring my MS by what I can still do and what I can no longer do. The gap that is created is where the pain of being ashamed resides. In situations where there was a gap, I would fill it with a massive dose of inadequacy. I thought of myself as less than I was. Shame was an unwanted acquaintance that seemed to settle in under my skin.

Being embarrassed along with being ashamed is a natural reaction to a life-altering and debilitating ailment such as MS. The disease certainly doesn't do me any favors, and the unknown future that is in store makes for a daunting reality. The biggest struggle with shame was early in my diagnosis when I was still trying to understand what was going on. I would have good days and bad days, but the bad days certainly had a greater impact on the way I saw myself. After a lifetime of mostly good days, I had taken so many of them for granted that I was not prepared to deal with the onslaught and degree of bad days that were now a certainty in my future.

Really for the first time in my life, I could say I truly knew what was meant by taking one step forward and two steps back. Sometimes I wouldn't see enough good days between the bad days in order to mentally heal. The unrelenting press put on by my MS wasn't playing fair and by the time another bad day would roll around, I was still feeling the shame from the last one. The situation was a vicious cycle that would leave me hanging my head and would cause my shoulders to slump.

Overcoming the feeling of being ashamed was not easy. I still have setbacks even to this day. They say you can only eat an elephant one bite at a time, and this is so very true for a personal sense of shame as well. I never believed for a second I would simply wake up one day and it would be gone...never to return. Like so many things I have dealt with having MS, I have taken bits and pieces back a little at a time. Ridding myself of feeling shame has been an incremental journey that requires keeping the realness of what shame can do front and center in my mind.

Even as I moved from understanding to accepting, I never underestimated the power and resiliency of feeling shame. While I have a much easier time now recovering from the feeling of being ashamed, I know it is even more important now to never allow my MS the opportunity to fill that gap. Even though I may not be able to do some of the things I could before MS, my sense of acceptance gives me the needed strength to fill the gap with something much better...something that sets me up to handle the good and bad days ahead.

Chapter 45: The Glass Is Never Half-Empty...Nor Half-Full

This is not meant to reference mental attitude or the notion of being an optimist or a pessimist. The notion behind this descriptive picture is related to one's outlook. Some people will look at the empty part of the glass while others will look at the filled part of the glass. In the context of acceptance, the glass must be looked at in its entirety. Acceptance is not a state of mind that is reached when only half-filled. There is no "almost there" measurement you can use. To admit you almost accept something is better said that you do not yet accept it.

As mentioned earlier in this section, one tends to move through a gray or shaded area between black and white from understanding to accepting. But at some point you definitively cross over and you know you are there. Acceptance lives and breathes with the one who possesses it. It is not fragile but rather takes the ups and downs with you as you move through life. It will become a friendly and calming force that you can call upon to see you through all that life will put in front of you.

Acceptance may take some people more time than others. I know for me it couldn't come fast enough. I was tested time and time again only to realize I wasn't there yet. Had I been, my actions and responses would have been different. They would have been more deliberate and constructive. MS can turn so many thoughts to negative emotions and resentment. Acceptance provides the strength to turn things around and get your emotions and actions back on a healthy and productive track.

If you have ever read the biography of Helen Keller, you will come to understand what true acceptance really means. This was a young lady who was without sight, hearing, or speech. Her life and struggle took her through understanding to accepting and ultimately accepting to overcoming. Yet she did not accomplish the things she was ultimately able to do without the complete transformation to total acceptance of her disabilities. It was here that she was able to turn her disabilities into abilities.

The glass of life will always have enough water to fill it. The question as to whether it is filled or not is better pictured as a glass with or without a hole in the bottom. If acceptance is not complete, then there is a hole in the bottom, and the water will drain out, leaving an empty glass. If acceptance is reached, then the glass will maintain all it was intended to hold. Point being, the glass can never be half-full.

Chapter 46: Managing the Symptoms

If there is one thing that makes having MS more difficult than other diseases or disorders, it is the symptomatic residue that is left behind by the damage the disease does. MS is certainly the cause of the symptoms, but with no cure most treatment paths that an MS patient will experience revolve around reducing symptoms. In fact, the disease itself acts in a rather silent environment, but the continual scarring or demylenation of nerve pathways can ultimately produce a variety of debilitating symptoms. It is the symptoms that ultimately take a toll.

Most of my damage at this point exists at the base of my brain and high up in my spinal column. This has resulted in a steady tremor in both my hands, along with significant loss of feeling in my upper extremities. At times, my symptoms can be painful as well as amplified. In the recent six months, I have also experienced increased symptomatic activity in my legs, particularly my right leg. While I have reduced sensitivity and feeling in both of my feet, my right leg doesn't always work as my brain is telling it to. Walking for me can appear clumsy and choppy. The other primary symptom I experience, and have for quite some time, is poor balance. Under most circumstances, it isn't bad enough to impact my walk or coordination, but there are times when it is very difficult to steady myself.

I have learned through my treatment that managing my symptoms is absolutely critical. Equally important is my ability to pay attention to my symptoms and to listen to what they are telling me. One of the worst things MS patients can do is ignore their symptoms, particularly when they become exacerbated. My doctor pays special attention to teaching his patients to listen to what your body is telling you. When you are overdoing it, your body will tell you. When stress is taking a toll, you can feel it. I certainly realize that under normal circumstances, overdoing it or stress (as an example) can cause a healthy person to experience symptoms. But when you have MS, it is much more pronounced. Many times, putting yourself in a difficult situation can stimulate symptomatic activity much more so than would ever be experienced by a person without MS.

One of the easiest things for me to overlook has been the need for ample rest. I have always been a person that has not needed much sleep to be able to function at relatively high levels of activity and accomplishment. If I would get six hours of sleep a night, I would wake up feeling pretty good and accomplish what the next day held in store. As time went on and MS entered my life, this was no longer the case. I may be able to make it two or three days with six hours of sleep, but at some point, I wouldn't be able to continue to function. I would have to take a long nap during the day or play catch up one night by packing in eight to ten hours.

The ability to read your body and respond to the symptoms accordingly is a big part of accepting this disease. I cannot deny my symptoms or pretend they will merely go away on their own. It will take active involvement and effort on my part to manage them. Even when my symptoms rob me of my effort or ability, I have to focus to the greatest degree on what has gotten me this far. I have to focus on

what I have come to accept and why. Like so many problems in life, I

have to find the path to manage it.

Chapter 47: Boundaries Merely Let You Know Where You Are

As my kids have gotten a little older, they always want to do more with their time. More sports, more fun, more adventure, more time to satisfy their curiosity and desires. Commitments that end up being made by them really are a family commitment. If they want to play a sport, it generally takes the family to understand and ultimately participate. If they want to go somewhere, it generally means further away from home for a longer period of time. It is not only fun for them, but it is a chance for the family to get centered and revitalized.

When you have MS, as much as you want to do these things with and for your family, it becomes much more difficult. The physical limitations experienced can not only be exhausting, they can downright stop you in your tracks. In time, these limitations end up having a mental impact on what you believe to be your boundaries, and you can put up a very high fence that keeps you locked inside. You can start to doubt yourself and think thoughts about letting down your family. If we go and do something, what will the kids think if dad can't make it? What will happen if he gets "sick"?

Boundaries held me back early in my MS. After my first relapse and really feeling the effect of my MS symptoms in an exponentially enhanced state, it really set me back on my heels. It made me give pause to just about everything I thought I could do. Could I watch my son practice or play a sport in the midsummer heat? Could I take an all-day attempt at an amusement park? I never liked the answers I would come up with, but there they were.

As I became more familiar with my MS and learned through acceptance to listen more closely to the disease, I started stepping out a little at a time and pushing the boundaries that I had built up. It was like setting an incremental goal every time I stepped out to do something. It usually took shape around my family. Maybe the kids wanted to go somewhere for spring break or we all decided to go one weekend and work on our farm; whatever it was, I tried to focus on doing more than I did the last time.

I began to see the boundaries not as the edge, but merely as a line to cross. Just as a marathon runner progressively trains to take on the entire marathon a little at a time, so would I. By managing my MS in this way, I could build my confidence, strength, and endurance one situation at a time. I didn't have to be worried about taking a huge jump in my physical capabilities because I was putting myself in situations that were manageable. In making them more manageable, I saw myself crossing the boundaries from before and gaining a step up on my MS.

While I realize that I have to be smart about things and not overdo it, this doesn't have to mean I simply succumb to what MS has made for my life. Even when it sets me back, I can come back...one situation at a time. Boundaries tend to be more of what we mentally make something out to be. Even when life does dish out something like MS, it is important to realize that boundaries are not walls; they are merely lines that we mentally draw, and with the right frame of mind, you can cross them. This is sometimes referred to as success in increments. Just as if you were to draw a circle around yourself, if you cross the line and face another line, you will soon realize that your circle is getting bigger. It is just like you were climbing a flight of stairs one step at a time. Soon, you will make it to the top.

Chapter 48: Watch the Road

When you are in high school it can feel like the world is waiting for you. Your future, college, your career, your future family; all of it is mysteriously unknown and exciting to think about. You assess your options and weigh what you want to do. Ultimately you make decisions to go a certain direction and so goes the rest of your life. It is much the same as most learn to assess options for other milestone choices to make as well. What will I major in? What job do I want to pursue? Who will I marry? What will I be like as a parent? All of these things fit nicely into the same decision tree for each of us.

What makes it so exciting is the fact that the road we take to get to these decisions leads to a litany of branches. All of these branches lead to a different place with yet more branches. Our uniqueness is not only rooted in our differing personalities, but the roads we choose to travel in life. Sometimes roads are placed in front of us unexpectedly and without the opportunity to make a choice. We may be "forced" to travel a particular road for a while, but it is important to realize that no road really comes to a dead end. No road comes without branches.

The road an MS patient will travel is no different; it comes with potholes, bumps, and obstacles which get in our way. Yet it also comes with branches. There will be a multitude of choices to make on this road, just as there are with any other road in life. To think it is a dead end or that there is no future opportunity to navigate is to close one's self off to the opportunity to choose. Not a good idea for any of life's milestones.

One of the reasons it is easy to fall into this frame of mind is the simple fact that it becomes quite easy with a disease such as MS to take your eyes off the road. It is easy to get distracted and lose sight of the road you are traveling. It is almost like traveling through a fog. You can become disoriented and not know what direction you are traveling or how fast you are going. Your mind begins to wander, and you begin to question yourself...am I even on the road anymore?

But if you work harder to remain focused, you can indeed collect your bearing. You have to look more intently at the landscape and peer through the fog. You call upon your senses and your mind to be tuned to your surroundings. It is really no different than when you lose your way in your career, or with the things that are truly important in your life. It can happen to any of us and does happen even to the best of us.

Watching the road is a skill that we hone over time. Just like experienced drivers, they will most certainly do it better than a beginner. I remember during my first relapse, I felt as if I was moving but couldn't really tell where the road was taking me. I lost track of getting better and became a clock watcher just waiting for someone to ring the bell and tell me it was over. I was more focused on what was behind me and couldn't see clear to what was in front of me. I was no longer sharp or aware of my surroundings. In a sense I was lost. But just like traveling on any stretch of road, you may hit a bump or pass by something familiar and you connect. For me, it was a time nearing the holidays and being around family helped to take my mind off watching the clock and got me back on track. You shake yourself awake and refocus on the road.

One thing is for certain, the road is long. It is windy and will take you up and down. It will take you by things familiar and other things you have never seen before. But when you place this road next to most others you will travel in life, it really isn't all that different. What makes the journey worthwhile, as hard as it may be, is one's ability to keep looking ahead and watch for what is coming. Paying attention will get you to another opportunity, and opportunity will mean a choice. No matter what decision you make, you will be the driver and not merely a passenger.

Chapter 49: Try Again

Throughout the trials and tribulations of learning about MS and what it was doing to my body, there were numerous events and situations that I can remember where I had to stop trying and accept the facts of my limitations. Early on in my diagnosis, there was a physical and mental reason for doing this. I wasn't sure about my limitations and what the consequences would be. I was inexperienced with dealing with my symptoms. Most of all, I had not come to terms with accepting my MS and the result of pushing myself would have been detrimental. To put it simply, I hadn't put in the time to relate to the action-reaction relation of doing the things I had prior to MS.

One of the most important activities that I believe has helped to define who I am has always been my ambition, skill, and interest in woodworking. Before MS, there was literally not one project that I took on that I was unable to complete. The personal satisfaction this provided was unmatched. Woodworking was where I began to see my MS limitations. With my perpetual tremor, I could not gain the

189

exactness nor approach the next step as I had always been able to do. I took this as failure and quite literally stopped trying for over a year.

As I moved from understanding to accepting, I started to realize how much I missed my passion. There had been a time when I remember talking to my wife about doing woodworking for a living. Before MS, I would have had no problem switching careers if I could have earned the living I was able to as compared to my current career. With MS, that thought initially seemed to only lead me to an improbable and maybe unattainable career option. As I reached deep down, I realized that my approach to woodworking wasn't all that different from my approach to MS. Sure I would have to think about my next step more intently…maybe I would even have to learn a new way to accomplish something…this was no different than how I would have to manage any woodworking project. Many of the projects I took on were first time efforts. So was my MS. Trying again somehow felt like the right thing to do; it felt natural.

I have gradually gotten back into the groove by taking on smaller projects and honing my skills. Sure I am different now. I know I am not the same "person" I was before MS and because of this, I will likely be unable to do the same things the same way I used to, but I do believe that eventually I will be able to do everything I once did. I feel the desire within me to take it on. I welcome the challenge and find myself laying in bed as I did before thinking about the next step to a project. I missed that for so long and wondered if I would ever get it back. The good news is my situation of overcoming and trying again can be the same for anyone with MS.

The will to do is contagious. I have always been a person who thrives on it. I can dream big again and know that so many things are possible. Learning the means to try something again is healthy for anyone. While everyone should face their shortcomings at some point in their life, there are a lot of folks I know who have never given themselves another chance. While it may sound counter-intuitive and even borderline-profound to admit, I am thankful for MS helping me to find my "do-over" spirit.

Chapter 50: The Building Blocks

There are a number of qualities that one could use to describe me, but I have generally been a person who does not spend much time proclaiming my qualities to others. In much the same way, I recollect a speaker at one of our company conferences that stated, "If you have to tell people you are a leader, then you are not." I have always believed it is better to show people your qualities over trying to convince people into believing you have them.

For me, I have learned through my dealings with MS, the important building blocks of life do not reside in the pursuit of material things. They do not reside in the proclamations I could make about myself. I have chased the trophies of our world and have succeeded in acquiring many of them, but not one of them helped me through this ordeal. Not one of them helped me through the perils of understanding or accepting my disease.

Journeying through a disease such as MS requires substantive qualities. It requires a physical and mental frame of mind that many will only realize in a time of desperation…just like I did. The trauma of what life can unveil can truly bring out the best of a person, and I firmly believe this "secret" has been revealed to me through my MS. These "best" qualities or building blocks reside in all of us. They are the force that cause us to reach deep down inside to find the means to our needed end. Without them, we are less than what we were intended to be.

I give credit to so many for placing these building blocks in front of me over my lifetime. My parents, wife and kids, sister, my wife's parents, friends and coworkers have all freely given whether known or unknown. These gifts are not found in the material world. You cannot purchase them. You do not earn them. They are a gift that you have to come to truly accept. But these building blocks are as real as any of the trophies of the world you may come to treasure. Not only are they as real…they are more. I was once asked the question, "Does God exist?" I remember answering this question with another question, "Do you love your family?" As many of us would state the answer to the question was, "Yes." My response was, "So if you love your family, then you would have to declare that love exists?" Again, as many of us would say, the answer was "Yes." Just as the answer to this question poses the same underlying meaning that I was asked, the real question was not necessarily intended to be answered if God or Love existed, but rather that there was proof behind an answer.

Building blocks actually confirm both. They show us and teach us to look within ourselves for the answer. While no one can prove through any of their actions, no matter how much they give or care or nurture that love "exists"; virtually all of us through our own human experiences know that it does. I can tell someone I love them. I can show someone I love them. But none of these actions on their own or in a cumulative fashion prove that love exists. Just as I cannot "prove" that God exists; I know that he does.

It is these same building blocks, the foundation of understanding and accepting, that I choose to invest. These are the true essence of living, regardless of the hand we are dealt. There is no regret. There is only joy. There is no disappointment. There is only sanctuary. When you have these building blocks, you will certainly stop looking for proof in the objects of the world and realize the proof comes from a much better place.

Part Three: Accepting to Beating MS

I remember being asked a question as a young adult that I recall made me stop and think long and hard about what it really meant. In fact the question was so compelling I remember even repeating it to myself, hoping that by doing so, I would somehow absorb the answer. The question was posed by a professor from the business school at the university I was attending. He asked, "What happens when an unstoppable force collides with an immovable object?"

I have reflected on this question many times over in my life since college, but no time as much as the past year. I don't know what the reason, other than a subconscious association of somehow personalizing the question for myself. Maybe I am the immovable object. Maybe my MS is the unstoppable force. In either the original question or my own mental fabrication, the meeting of the two makes for an almost unimaginable result. I never would have thought about an immovable object meeting an unstoppable force if it were not for that college professor. Of course, I would never have imagined myself encountering MS either.

While I realize I am not an immovable object nor is MS an unstoppable force, the analogy appropriately fits for this final section. The likeness in my personalized analogy seems to come down to one common thread for me...respect. I have a great deal of respect for myself and my responsibilities to myself and my family. I have a great deal of respect for my MS, just as I would any worthy opponent. As I reflect on the qualities I know are ever so important to me, I become that unmovable object. As I realize there is no cure for MS today, it becomes the unstoppable force.

This analogy is not intended to be drawn to the likeness of a comic book hero who fights the evils of the world to always and ultimately prevail. Nor is it intended to portray some unattainable reckoning that none of us can relate to. In stark contrast, we all can come to a similar crossroads in our lives. We can all end up in a place where we are so driven to get to where we want to go, and yet it seems like there is the existence of a perpetual obstacle that stands in our way. This is where we make our stand. This is where I intend to plant my feet and answer the question my college professor posed to me over twenty years ago.

Chapter 51: Make Plays to Win

I have to think before I act. There is a great deal more preparation in setting out to do things than before. In the days before MS, it would be nothing for me to step outside and work for hours in the yard or take up a woodworking project in the garage and stay at it all night. Not so anymore. It isn't that I can't do these same things, but there is significantly more planning and time involved beforehand, during, and after.

Thinking before acting is solid advice for anyone. This point though is not intended to be oversimplified. The thinking I am referring to involves playing a game of chess, not checkers. There are always the obvious and basic actions that seem to come natural in thought. Actions tend to almost become automatic. The thinking involved in making decisions around my MS is much more strategic than before. It is more deliberate. Listening to your body is an invaluable trait when you have MS, but being prepared and able to think your way through what you can expect from an action before you are in the situation, is a winning move that compliments paying attention to what your body is telling you.

Setting myself up for a successful action is no accident. It is not up to someone else to make this happen. I own it. It builds character and confidence. It breeds satisfaction and the ability to think myself to wider circles. Making plays founded in this way of thinking is essential to a healthy mind and body.

I used to think that my dad always thought about things too much. He never seemed to be spontaneous enough for me. Even now, he is a very deliberate man, assessing most moves he makes well before he acts on them. Yet now that I find myself thinking more and more like him as it relates to my actions, I see the wisdom in his approach. While I admit I haven't quite lost all of my spontaneity, particularly when it comes to decisions involving money, I have matured with my MS to set myself up for a win against this disease someday.

Making plays to win, thinking myself through to an action, becomes as constant and steady as breathing. Whether at work or at play, whether in my own yard or a thousand miles from home, my thoughtfulness in setting myself up for a worthwhile action, seeing myself through all the tasks involved, and reflecting after to know what I need to do better the next time, have become a valiant weapon in my fight. Mistakes in my actions only prove I am human. But making the choice to play chess in life instead of checkers proves that I can still overcome even with MS; I can play to win.

Chapter 52: Setbacks Will Happen

As much as I try to stay clear of a relapse or aggravating symptoms, the fact is that MS is still a disease that progresses to do damage to my nervous system. The reality of this cannot be confused with a lack of effort on my part to do everything I can to ensure it is mitigated and kept in check. Despite the effort though, MS will open the door and let itself in. I have to expect it. Relapses will happen and the damage will progress throughout my life; it is inevitable.

When a setback happens, there are several fundamental things I have to remind myself. They are actually fairly simple, and when followed, they immensely help. It all centers on turning to the things that work. One, control your environment as much as possible. With my particular sensitivity to heat, I have to stay away from it during a setback. Others may have dominant symptoms that they will come to learn what helps and what hurts. Sticking with what helps during a setback is critical. Two, I have to give myself time to recover. My first relapse took weeks for me to really get back to being myself.

There was no rushing it. Just like a broken bone needs time to heal, so does my body. Three, I get with my doctor as soon as possible for follow up and treatment. The treatment paths my doctor follows have proven to be extremely beneficial for expediting recovery. I can't say to myself I will wait a few days and see if things get better; this would be a huge mistake for me. When I know that a setback or relapse has happened, I do not wait. It becomes a number one priority to get in to my doctor.

There are also the mental aspects of working through setbacks. With acceptance, I learned that setbacks are a part of having MS and there is no denying them. But I can see myself past it. Keeping a positive attitude is hard as it would be for most people, but a trained mind can give you the insight you need to look beyond the setback and keep you moving past it.

Another reality of MS setbacks is the innumerable people in my life that truly want to help. Help has always meant weakness for me personally if I was to accept it, but since MS, I have learned that I need to welcome it. Accepting help from others does not mean I am weak, in fact; it shows my strength of acceptance. There are a lot of great people out there who genuinely want to help. My wife is one such person for me, and there are many others in my life.

Whether I am at the beginning, middle, or end of a setback, I take seriously to learning from the experience. Because of the way MS works, it will talk to me. It will reveal what it is doing. It has been helpful for me to keep a journal to chronicle my symptoms, thoughts, doctor visits, treatments, what worked and what did not. Over time, I can look back and my notes seem to make more sense. The puzzle pieces fit together much easier.

I try to see setbacks as merely a part of life. There are even the setbacks that have nothing to do with MS. If I focus on the setback as simply a part of my life and not merely a part of having MS, then it doesn't seem to feel so unique to the disease. While these setbacks will most certainly happen to me, including the setbacks related to my

MS, I will not let shame and doubt enter in. I am better prepared for the next one that comes along and better prepared to get through it.

Chapter 53: Encouraging Will Over Want

Remember what it is like to want something so much it ends up consuming most of your thoughts and efforts? No matter what you do or think, the desire creeps into your every move and slowly turns your thinking so that the want is front and center. You did it when you were a child, and you do it as an adult. Sure the wants are very different, but the desire to want remains as childlike as it was when you were young. It is a basic and essential trait we all possess that helps us to dream, desire, and wish.

But what generally happens when all we do is "want" after something? Do we usually get it? I know for me, it usually doesn't work this way. I can want something or want an event to happen so much that I can almost taste it, but that doesn't make it come to reality. I can spend hours, days, or even weeks in want of something, and it tends to remain as distant as when my initial thought produced it.

It is not that wanting is a bad thing. But wanting is a passive activity. By itself it goes nowhere. If all we had to do to get something was merely want to get it, then all of our lives would definitely be very different. I would want my MS to go away and let the forces of my desires play themselves out to make it happen. Nothing is that easy. As the saying goes, "There is no such thing as a free lunch." Wanting can ignite action, but I like to believe that it turns into something much more before anything of substance can really happen. I can want something to happen, and at times this is where it starts, but it has to turn from a "passive" to an "active" activity. The things of substance and fiber we want for ourselves will require clear thought and effort. The spark for this to occur happens when we turn our want into will. Willing for something is very different. It is that point that we turn to actionable thought. To will something to happen goes so much deeper than a want that merely resides on the surface. Will turns a wish into hope. It turns a desire into a goal.

Think of it in terms of the election process. If everyone merely wanted their candidate to win, but no one voted, what would happen?

The will of the people moves them to vote for their candidate of choice, and this action makes the goal of seeing their candidate win a reality. This result could not happen any other way. This is the essential difference between wanting and willing.

Fighting MS has been a will-driven battle. I have left wanting it to go away, right next to dreaming about it going away. They are both short-lived and disappointing in the end. Instead, I will myself to deal with it, and through this I am able to fight behind a mindful plan laden with goals and expected accomplishments. Insight and effort become so clear, I end up realizing myself to a larger circle of opportunity, breeding more will and the process continues to repeat itself. When my next relapse happens, my spark will be my will. When I accomplish completing the remodel of our farmhouse despite my MS, willing it across the finish line will be behind the entire effort.

Willing something over wanting something makes all the difference. Realizing there is a difference happened for me, and it can happen for you.

Chapter 54: I'm Worth It

How much value do we place on the things around us? Our home, family, job, even our bank account all have value to us. We tend to naturally think of "value" or "worth" for the objects in our lives in terms of their monetary measure. How much money we have or how much is my investment worth simply means how much money would it yield if I were to sell it. Other more important things in our lives, at least they should be more important, such as friends and family have a natural course for measurement as well. We tend to look at worth or value from the perspective of what these individuals give us and how they make us feel. We may take inventory of what they have done for us, how much they seem to love or care for us, or how dependable they may be.

Value and worth of the animate and inanimate objects in my life have changed over time, as I'm sure they do for a great deal of people. It is not so much that the nature of these things have changed, for instance, I know for certain my parents have always loved me, but the value I have placed on them has changed as I have matured and gone through various phases of my life. What they were "worth" in my mind when I was sixteen is very different than what they are "worth" today. As my perspective on life has changed and grown, so has the value I place on things around me.

I have always thought of myself as a fairly good person, but I have known deep down for many years that I could have done more for people and for the various situations that I have been in. I'm not sure that it was my encounter with MS that enlightened me or a combination of MS and other people or events. Whatever it was, I know that through my process of understanding and accepting my MS, there was solidification in my outlook on what things were worth. The outlook is entirely fresh for me and provides for possibilities that I would have never been able to foresee through my prior value assessment approach.

This change in my view has shifted to the idea that worth is a measurement based on the power of contribution. In this way, I don't think of the inanimate objects in a way that would require me to sell or somehow convert them into a monetary means to an end. My job is not simply the value of my paycheck. My house is not worth only what I could sell it for. Rather, the worth of these resides in the way they contribute to my life and my family. My job gives us the ability to do so many things. It provides the resources not only for us to live, but also to experience the joys of life. Our house is not simply an investment that someday we hope to make money on, but rather contributes to our having a home and a place to make memories, grow and become closer.

By applying this to people, the power of value and worth becomes almost limitless. Not only do I assess the joy or experience interacting with someone may give me and the ability these feelings and knowledge may provide for me, but this way of thinking invariably draws me to assess myself. What I am worth is not rooted in how much money I make or what I own. It is not rooted in how much money I can draw out of my checking account or what I can buy. It is founded in what I can give.

Admitting I am worth it is not a statement of arrogance as one might imagine. It is a peaceful understanding I have that is simply based on my belief that I have the power to contribute tomorrow more than I did today. If I can be a better husband and father, a better friend and coworker, then the value and worth I can help create will never need to have a price tag placed on it. What would our relationships and outlook on life be like if we all valued things in this way…starting with ourselves? I beat MS a little more every day because of this outlook. The power of my contribution can be so much more than that of this disease, and through this, I know I am valuable. I know I am worth it.

Chapter 55: Inclined for Greatness

Have you ever thought about what you were truly meant to do in life? I know we think about it probably hundreds of times throughout our lives and maybe always arrive at a variety of answers. I recall when I was young, it was common for adults to ask this question whether it was a teacher in school or a relative on a visit. Their question would be posed with an unassuming ascent of eagerness for an answer, "What do you want to do when you grow up?" The question seemed so much simpler to answer back then. I remember always having a list that comprised my response.

I see myself more fortunate than most as my life has carried on, and I have had the privilege to live out the reality of this question by being able to pursue most anything I thought I was meant to do. My grandfather used to remind me there are people in this world that do not get to choose certain things for themselves, including what they will be. Even living in a country as great as ours with so many unlimited opportunities, this same question is not all that easy to answer. I not only have wrestled with what I was going to do with my life, but how I was going to do it would also pose many challenges.

In life there are so many outside forces that can turn things upside down. There are accidents and tragedies, there is crime and poverty, and then there is illness and death that make the notion of living...much less how to live...near impossible at times. I honestly do not recall feeling so insecure about my life, how I was going to live it, and what I was going to do with it, as I did when I learned I had MS. The hardest time was before my diagnosis and then shortly thereafter. I did not understand it, and I definitely had not accepted it. I searched and searched for the answer to the question of what I was meant to do with MS, but the answers just would not present themselves to me.

MS took the wind out of my sail. If it wasn't bad enough to end up with MS, I also had the compounded problem of now wondering what it would allow me to do with my life. The question has never been more real for me until then. I had always found a reason to hold back from doing what I really believed I should be doing, but that was a decision I had made. I was in control of my direction in life. My reasons always seemed like good reasons. They were always the responsible thing to do. While I certainly do not regret the decisions I have made of what to do with my life, I have always known I could be doing more. But again it was always my decision. Now I had MS; how was I going to get there now?

If I had not changed my outlook on my diagnosis, I'm certain I would still be asking that same question today. As I came to understand and then accept my MS, I noticed my thoughts about what I could and should be doing with my life began to change. I started seeing myself no longer holding back from what I could become. I started to realize that I had a responsibility to go beyond all that I had conservatively reasoned to do in life…and now do it with MS.

I have worked with my family on remodeling an entire house for over two years now. From bare studs up to a finished home inside and out, we are doing it all by ourselves. The first year of the project,

I was extremely symptomatic, frustrated, and did not know what was going on. But something kept me going. The second year, I had been diagnosed, and while things went slower than I had wanted, we had now progressed to almost completing the remodel. Within another six months or so, the house will be complete. I have never been more convicted to do this in my life than I am right now with MS. And still something keeps me going.

I am convinced that we are all here to do great things. We simply have to be inspired to do them. MS has helped to ignite my drive to not hold back with what I should be doing with my life. I am ready to answer the question if anyone were to ask it again with the same eagerness they did when I was a child. Greatness is not necessarily measured by accomplishment, but rather by overcoming the struggle to get there. MS doesn't have to keep you from greatness. In fact, it may even help you get there.

Chapter 56: The Individuality of MS

One of the medical facts that has been very interesting about MS is that while the disease attacks the central nervous system in all those that have it, MS shows itself through symptoms that are quite different depending on the patient. In part, this is certainly due to the damage and where in the nervous system the damage resides. But even when the damage is in a similar part of the brain or spine, for two different patients it will likely not show itself as similar symptoms. In speaking with my doctor as he has elaborated on this subject in several of our discussions, it just goes to show how much we still have to learn about this disease. Maybe it is due to age, maybe gender, or maybe the timing of where a person is in the disease state, any of these things and certainly other factors, makes MS very unique to every individual that has it.

MS seems to tailor itself differently to each of its hosts. In an almost designer-like fashion, MS eludes any consistency in damage or result. Some people may show very large lesion activity on their MRI, but their symptoms are relatively light, while others show smaller lesion activity on their MRI, but their symptomatic activity is heavy and pronounced. My lesions tend to be smaller, but my symptomatic activity can greatly swing and show itself in very pronounced ways.

While on the surface this fact about MS can lead anyone afflicted by this disease to utter and sheer frustration, I have learned that it does point me in a particular direction as an understanding and accepting patient. The unpredictability and individuality of MS can become a weapon in your favor. There are a number of therapeutic options that may not work for others, but could be an extremely viable solution for me or you. Don't rule them out just because you know other MS patients have had less than promising results. That matters not to your own individual MS.

The individuality MS breeds across an array of patients will tend to foster a strong internal drive to individualize your response. I believe a good portion of the success I have had dealing with my MS has been based in knowing the tailored nature of my MS and relying on my individual effort to listen to what MS is doing to me...not necessarily to others...and then responding to my MS with my own tailored response. If it works, file it away as a success, and keep it close at hand. Learn from it, grow from it, and use it the next time you have to figure things out.

Individuality is a great trait to possess. While it makes MS a bit trickier to deal with, it can make you a bit trickier with a response. I do not see the inconsistency MS presents to the patient population as a reason to be inhibited. While MS may have the characteristics of individuality, it is not near as powerful as the individuality of a person or the individuality of a person's potential. History has shown what we can accomplish through the strength of our individuality. As we grow as individual contributors to ourselves, our family, and our community; we can make the impossible turn to possible. In time, the same will shine through in our individual battles with MS.

Chapter 57: The Value of Time

Time seems to be that elusive event in which we live that never goes fast enough when we are young and never goes slow enough as we get older. Time runs the cogs in the wheel that creates the canvas by which a plethora of situations and circumstances shape what we ultimately call our life. No amount of money can purchase it. When it is gone, you cannot get it back, and how much lies ahead of each of us is certainly unknown. And yet like most of us, I have valued it based mostly on what time in my life has already been spent. The value that time has for me is mentally measured based on what I was able to do with it…what I was able to create and accomplish. I never really took the time (pardon the pun) to value the time in my future, whether it ends up being only one more day or fifty more years. It doesn't really matter how much of it remains. It only comes down to the value I prospectively will place on it.

During my diagnosis phase, all the time I recall dating back to my first symptoms to the time right up to and soon after my diagnosis,

I was like the child where time couldn't go fast enough. I wanted to get to the next "event". Maybe then I would know what this was all about. It was well before understanding and accepting MS in my life, and while I mentally mark the time during this period as frustrating and depressing…certainly not well spent…I realize now I should have had more tenacity and fortitude to apply more effort and value in it.

The biggest regret I have in my reflection is why did I not do more with that time? At any rate, I'm not going to waste any more of it thinking what I could or should have done. My focus is to move on and look to proactively value the time in my future in a very different way. I'm worth it. My family is worth it. My time is certainly worth it.

I don't believe I would be able to have such a positive outlook on the value of time in the wake of such a devastating disease had it not been for my maturity to understand and accept my future with MS. Time is not the enemy. It will continue to lay life's canvas in front of me with or without this disease. I know that now and embrace it with the tenacity and fortitude I wish I had before. The cogs in the wheel may stop at any time, but I will not stop my living short of that fact.

This is a great lesson I can now take to all aspects of life's intended efforts. While MS has been painted on my canvas, so too have other things that are great. MS is marked by shades of gray, but the great things are marked with vibrant and bold colors. They all aid in painting my picture of life. These events that create the color over time begin to complement each other and will come together to make my life's story. Valuing the time it takes to accomplish this, including all the strokes that will take place in the future, will ultimately mean the difference between just a picture and a masterpiece. I choose the masterpiece.

Chapter 58: Honor the People Placed Around You

I have referenced a number of individuals, particularly in Part One, that have had a profound impact not only on my life in general but particularly on my life with MS. From my wife to my boss, my parents to teammates, my in-laws to distant siblings; all have provided an immeasurable network of support that has helped me through the tumultuous journey of MS entering my life. They all have left such a positive impression on me that it has changed me forever.

I remember years after I graduated college and married my wife, we had a conversation about old high school and college friends. She used to be a person who referred to everyone she knew or referenced in conversation as a "friend". Our discussion was a mutual reflection of what it meant to be a friend and if these people were really deserving of such a title? As I took inventory myself, I was shocked to come to the realization that there was not one person from my high school or college life that I would call at this time a "friend". Not that it was their fault; I was just as guilty for not staying in touch or showing interest in their lives. Yet the truth of the situation was that not one of them knew much about me or vice versa. It was depressing to admit it, but nonetheless the truth.

Sometimes the natural coasting in life can lead to complacency toward others, and that is exactly what happened to me. Maybe it was the distance or span of time that contributed to the end result, but I know now what I missed by not paying more attention to the people placed in my early adult life, and I have genuine regret for allowing such a lapse to occur. People are precious cargo that we can choose to allow onboard our journey or leave on the curb as we pull away. We won't really know how valuable having them along could have been until we break down and are stranded.

MS was at first a breakdown in my life. I was stranded in the middle of a barren stretch of road. Fortunately for me, I had people that were traveling with me. They were resourceful, encouraging, and genuine givers of themselves. There are not many things in my life to date that I cannot imagine not accomplishing on my own, except for my battle with MS. I know that without these individuals, I would likely still be stranded in the middle of that distant road. They have not only helped me to change, but they have helped me to change my perspective on what it means to be a "friend".

I actually look forward to the next time my wife and I talk about the same topic we discussed nearly fifteen years ago; I know my thoughts and conclusions on the matter will be very different. Even my wife has changed her reference to what people mean in her life. If you happen to earn the title of "friend" in her life, I know that it is a deserved position she honors. She doesn't take it lightly, and through my battle with MS, I wholeheartedly agree with her today.

Don't let it take a disease such as MS to teach you what the people placed in front of you really mean. I learned the lesson the hard way…but I learned it all the same. People are placed in front of us for a reason, and it is up to each of us to find a way to be that person for others in need. I'm not afraid to travel the road of MS anymore because of the cargo I carry. The people who are there for me, I will always refer to as a "friend" for life and what they mean to me I will

honor for the rest of my time.

Chapter 59: Finish the Things You Start

This is obvious advice for anyone, but is something that I know I have taken for granted over the course of my life. There have been countless things, whether small or big, that I have not completed when I should have. It is more clearly understood when we are younger, as our attention spans are shorter, and we simply lose interest in what we were intent on doing. Yet as we mature, the incompleteness that we leave as a result of unattended closure creeps into our subconscious, and no matter how much we may come to reason why we maybe didn't finish something, it starts to grind on us.

The grinding can turn into guilt which might not be all that bad if it changes our outlook on finishing what we start. On the other hand, the grinding can lead to complacency which can quickly turn in to laziness and pretty soon we can find ourselves starting and not finishing so much in life. If we are completely honest with ourselves, the grinding in the very least forces us to a state of disappointment towards ourselves. No matter our station in life, it is a lump-in-the-throat sensation that is very difficult to swallow.

I have considered myself rather fortunate, as for most of my adult life, I have not been riddled with guilt when I start something and find myself contemplating not finishing it. I may not have wanted to finish it, but I likely did. Granted in many of these types of situations, my finishing touches were probably not as enthusiastic or productive as they would have been had I truly desired to bring things to closure in the right frame of mind. When my life was introduced to MS, I was even more concerned that I would have yet another easy reason to not finish things. After all, if I got to that point, I could easily chalk it up to MS as the reason I was unable to finish it.

Yet ailments such as MS can also bring out the best in people. I have heard stories from people with MS who are doing things now that they probably never would have started, much less completed, before they had MS. People have completed marathons and triathlons. Others have gone skiing for the first time and have made it a yearly adventure. Some have even gone back to school and started new careers. All because of the turning point of MS in their lives.

I have noticed that I have a stronger desire to start and finish things now. While I might be more careful in what I assume I am able to do, I seem more committed when I have made my mind up to pursue a goal or effort. Not only do I have more drive to get to my intended result, I maintain more focus throughout the effort. Even when I am not successful in my result, I know that my effort was genuine, and the guilt of quitting or not closing things out never creeps in. I am more satisfied with myself despite the outcome.

There seems to be a dormant spark within each of us that can turn us in to something more than we were when it is ignited. Conviction and tenacity stand in the wings of our efforts waiting for us to take hold and use them. I know that I will not be able to finish things to my liking every time. But I also know that I will not have regrets. Life and the things to do in life are too important to start and not finish. The spark that we all need to find can come from that

231

which we least expect. It may even come from something that we would have assumed would never give anything back. Even though MS has served up lemons, it has also helped me to find a way to make lemonade.

Chapter 60: Find Your Freedom

Freedom is a word often taken for granted. The founding of our country was based on the pursuit of freedom, at the cost of thousands of lives. Since even that time, it has cost thousands more. The world pursues it. We long for the result of freedom, but so many times we do not have the means to begin to take it on. Freedom is elusive and to so many whimsical. For some, it is like the comic-book hero one can only read about but later come to realize may not exist. Whether freedom is based in reality or in a comic-book-like setting, many of us reach out for it at some point in our lives.

My father served in Vietnam. He was a military officer at a time when the United States saw freedom in the world at the brink of collapse. He didn't write policy nor enact it. He saw his duty to defend it and was called upon by his country to fight for it. He doesn't talk about it much, and regretfully I haven't thanked him for his commitment to such a noble cause, but nonetheless he is a hero not only to this nation for his service, but also to me as a son and benefactor of his actions.

Freedom is not free. Whether in a war-torn effort or sitting in modern day America, one must realize this. Freedom has always had a price on it and it is always earned. Some struggles for freedom resonate even in our own country, despite the founding of our nation, and continue even to this very day. Yet the battle, regardless of the basis, is rooted in a struggle of pure release. It is a pursuit from that which binds us. Founded in the right to choose, freedom provides the medium by which we can decide.

When you look at the modern era, or back in history a thousand years, freedom has never been something given or granted. To reach a true state of freedom whether individually or as a nation it has only been realized through persistent effort and diligence. It is worth dying for. At the same time, it is worth fighting to live for. Freedom offers so much it is even hard to truly define. One thing is for certain, freedom possesses the qualities of life that so many of us use to quantify the value of our own personal and societal efforts. Whether in battle to defend a nation or a battle to beat a personal enemy, finding freedom is generally the measuring stick used to determine who will be named the victor.

Through my personal battle with MS, I have often thought about what freedom means to me. Maybe as bits and pieces have been taken away from me by MS, I have come closer to realize what freedom really means. While freedom has generally been defined by the actions and on the backs of so many from an historical context, I have come to know the notion of freedom in a much more personal sense. While I never served my country as my father did to fight for freedom in the traditional sense, I realized that I was involved in an intense battle against something that had the capability of stripping me of something very similar.

Finding your freedom is not a passive act. It is a struggle…a battle…a significant fight. It will break you down but can build you up. As a noted general once said during the American Revolution,

"War is first won in your mind and then carried out in your actions." For what would freedom really mean to any of us if it were not for something we had to struggle to achieve? Freedom is truly a search. Whether individually or as a nation, freedom provides the bounty by which we all have the chances we deserve.

I have known so many assumed freedoms in my life that the very word has been taken for granted. Yet MS has forced me to accept the notion of freedom in a whole new context. Freedom has helped me to wake up each and every morning longing for its benefit. The very definition of freedom expands because of the attention I give it. I know that MS has the power to keep me from realizing it, and what it means to me conjures up a strength that I didn't know I had. I am a fighting machine because of what freedom really means to me now. While so many have fought and died for freedom's defining moments, why would I do anything less for myself.

Chapter 61: Live a Simple Life

I don't know why life seems to end up so complicated at times. Maybe it's the world around me or maybe it's me and the way I have chosen to deal with the world. Whatever the reason, it is certain for most of us, it can end up this way over time. Complexity seems to abound for most facets of life. Illness only adds to it. The intertwining of people and living out life generally entails getting past complex problems and obstacles with the desired end result leaving us better off. Where I have most often fallen short is trying to deal with the complexities of life with complex solutions. Sometimes they work and sometimes they don't.

MS is in fact a complex disease. While there is much today that has been learned about MS from a scientific standpoint, there remains no cure. The cause of MS eludes us all, and yet hundreds of thousands of people, in this country alone, have had MS thrust upon them to make their lives even more complex to figure out. I have tried to do everything I can to overcome the impact of MS in my life, but more times than not when I have tried to present a complex solution to the problem, I have ended up disappointed.

I am not saying that everything should be simple or that every solution will be simple to achieve. Rather I have been more successful dealing with the complexities of life including my MS when I take a simpler approach. This doesn't mean I am not prepared or that the effort is any less. In fact, I find that when I center myself in simplicity, I am able to focus more attentively, execute more clearly and not allow MS to invade the epicenter of my life.

If I look at my parents who recently retired in the past few years, I can see the same concept at work. For most of us, we envision retirement as a time of getting back to the basics. We see ourselves doing things we have long forgotten or been unable to do because of other complex issues surrounding making a living and raising a family. We plan for the day when we will be able to relax and return to the simpler priorities of life such as travel, spending time with grandchildren, or even checking off the litany of items on our bucket list.

Living a simpler life though doesn't have to wait until retirement. In fact, it shouldn't. This is such a primal need we all have; it seems a bit ridiculous that we would wait until we are in the waning years of life to actually start to do it. Aside from the aging factor, other facts of life can also draw us to a simpler living philosophy, and MS has done this for me. I do not underestimate the disease. I know it is difficult, debilitating, and only intends to rob me of life's pleasure. But I believe it is expecting me to approach it with an arsenal of complex retaliation. Instead, I have thrown it a curve ball. I work to maintain a clear and simple perspective on what is truly important. Courage, positive attitude, family, and living the "retired" life, now leave my MS in the rearview mirror.

I look back and chuckle at how wrapped up I would get in trying to live through an artificial and complicated list of disguised priorities. And I did all of this without MS! Simple living has meant as much to me and my health as any medical treatment could provide. I know what MS can do to me, and I know that the progression of the disease will likely take a physical toll on me over time. But I can smile everyday because I clearly see how much more there is to simply living. In this way I have come to value living through a new lens. Through the lens of a simpler life and a simpler way of approaching it, MS loses its foothold, and the brightness of life's true intentions for me prevails.

Chapter 62: The Essence of Winning

There are hundreds of famous athletes and even more scholarly and accomplished people who have provided their take on the essence of winning. They all have their own commentary on the matter, and I will not dare to take anything away from what they believe this concept to mean. Yet all of them speak from their own experiences whether rooted in victory or in defeat. Their conclusions are deeply seeded in what winning has done for them and to them.

The basis of winning seems to be founded in the concept of a zero sum "game". In this game, there exists a winner as well as a loser. You cannot have one without the other. All sporting events to military incursions are measured in this manner. To define the winner means to also define the loser. To define it any other way would take away from both. People throughout history have relied on this concept as a way to associate their feelings, efforts, and skills to an end result. The result is never certain nor is the relationship established to the result for anyone involved until the winner and loser are determined.

When I think back on my fight against MS, it started off as a stacked deck against me. I was certain that I would lose. I did not understand the disease very well. I did not have the winning qualities to see victory through to the finish. I was convinced that if I engaged in the "game", it would spell certain defeat. But just like any winning athlete or military strategist, I needed to start off learning my opponent. To know what I would be up against was essential. There was no cutting corners or quick reference guide to bank on. I had to know how to play the game in order to know how to win.

From learning and knowing how to play the game, I then had to envelope an instinctive ability to act and react to the way MS would play the game. This couldn't be based on luck or some other haphazard action. It would have to be very deliberate, and I would have to be ready. Winning against MS could not be left to chance. Understanding the disease meant I knew what I was up against. I knew the consequences of a flawed effort.

If knowing is half the battle, then the other half is rooted in execution. Once I engaged MS, there was no turning back. There has been no timeout, halftime, or seventh-inning stretch in this game. It is an all-out battle to the end. The end will define the winner and the loser.

MS is formidable, but I have become formidable as well. The game is on, and we will see what happens when an immovable object meets an unstoppable force. They say winners can see the victory play out in their head before it happens. I play this out in my mind every day; I see myself a winner against MS, and it consumes my effort to be better than it is.

As each day goes by, I apply what I learn to be a better opponent against MS. My understanding and accepting this disease turns into believing more and more in my abilities and skills to beat it. I take the fight seriously and will never underestimate the next move I will have to make. I know I will win. No one who was victorious started off seeing themselves as the loser. They all knew they could do it. They found a way to associate their feelings, effort, and skills to the result they believed in. Through this they discovered the essence of winning, and so will I.

Chapter 63: Waking to Another Day

There have been many mornings since my diagnosis; not as many though as those that likely lay ahead. I reflect back on those mornings where I would wake up and lie still almost believing for a moment that maybe it is gone. I have learned a lot, and I have experienced even more. There have been good days and there have been bad days. Just like for most of us, the time for me has gone by quickly thinking back on it all. At times I still worry about things. I still wonder what MS will mean to me in five, ten or even twenty years.

MS has changed things in and around me forever. Amazingly, most of what has changed has been the choices I have made regarding reincorporating myself back into life and not so much what MS has done to me. For a while, MS made my world very dark. If you have never been in complete darkness, it is an eerie feeling. I remember walking deep into an extinct lava tube in Maui and turning off my light. The darkness was so thick; it engulfed me. It is so saturating and empty it almost feels like the space around you has become cemented blackness. There is a feeling of hopelessness, insecurity, and the unknown. You long for anything that can provide a sense of perspective and vision. This tomb that MS placed me in seemed impossible to escape and likely does for other MS patients as well.

Others came into the darkness to help me through it, but it was still my darkness. No matter what they did, whether it was medical help or family and friends providing their own light to help guide me, I had to realize that the darkness would not go away without finding that which was inside me to be a sustainable light. I would have to reach down inside myself like I had never done before to find it. My boss recently sent me a quote that in many ways sums up this journey that lay ahead of me, "It's what you learn after you know it all that counts." Unfortunately, I could not rely on all that I knew or thought I knew to produce the light. I would have to learn something new and make it count.

And so began my journey that I have tried to capture through this book. While I stood in my darkness from MS, I was able to find that something of sustainability...something that would light my way. A candle does not seem to produce much light when you are standing with it out in the sunshine, but in total darkness even the smallest light, even that from a single candle, can be so bright it finds its way through even the hardest blackness. This light is living and must be nurtured and once found, it will show the way.

It is made with patience, self reliance, determination, perseverance, inspiration, and then wrapped with courage, truth, and dignity. MS may have provided a darker world around me, but I have a brighter light by which to navigate. I don't think I would have ever found it without that darkness. For this fact I am truly grateful.

Now I look forward to each day seeing the light. The void of MS does not define me. The light pushes it back a little more every time I feed it and follow through with its intended purpose. This purpose is the true essence of living...even with MS. My light shines despite a worthy opponent. It grows with me and reveals new and exciting things. The light comes through the window, penetrating and filling the room, as I awake to another day.

www.ingramcontent.com/pod-product-compliance
Lightning Source LLC
Chambersburg PA
CBHW060242290526
45789CB00001B/158